GOOD MEDICINE

GOOD MEDICINE

A Return to Common Sense

Carol L. Roberts, M.D.

MERCURIUS PRESS

MERCURIUS PRESS

ISBN: 978-0-9779316-2-0

Library of Congress Control Number: 2009934117

PRINTED IN THE UNITED STATES OF AMERICA

Acknowledgements

First and foremost, I want to acknowledge the influence of my loving parents. They wanted, more than anything, for me to have a good education and to be able to take care of myself. They would be proud, I think, to know that I take care of others as well.

The information in this book comes from a thirty-plus year experience in clinical practice—in surgery, in the ER, and finally in the field of integrative/holistic medicine.

The examples of my professors were incorporated into my practice style. I thank them for their patience, their humor, and their generous sharing of what they know.

The experience of treating patients—both successfully and not—led to a constant search for gentle alternatives to conventional harsh and risky treatments. The practitioners who contributed to my learning were many—doctors, nurses, nutritionists, acupuncture physicians, homeopaths, naturopaths, astrologers, body workers, sound therapists, Reiki practitioners, and medical intuitives (you know who you are). They gave generously of their wisdom so that I could see what treasures lay outside the black bag. They loved that I wanted to know. I love and respect them for their persistence in swimming upstream, and for their love and respect for their clients.

Thanks to my staff, who are the backbone and the muscle of our clinic, Wellness Works. They do their jobs with patience and good humor in spite of all efforts to derail and discombobulate them. Amazing people, all of them.

Most of all, I want to thank the patients through the years, in all my various incarnations as a doctor, who allowed me to "practice" on them. Their feedback, their appreciation of my efforts, and their love sustain the uphill swim. In the end it will have been worth the trouble, for the smile on their faces and their delight in being free of illness, back to life, and in the swim at last. Of course, they are then automatically deputized as ambassadors of wellness to the remainder of the population, who still suffer under the "for-profit" industry which is conventional medicine.

And thanks to the Creator who gave me this job, this calling, this mission, that has made my time in Earth School so interesting and totally worth the trip.

ꙭꙭꙭꙭ

The cover art is by gifted watercolorist Sigrid Tidmore. The image depicts the famous medical symbol, the caduceus, in an updated form. The "new" medical symbol is vital, fierce yet fragile and vulnerable at the same time. It is thoroughly alive, just as medicine can become a living responsive system again that pays respect to all the natural world.

Contents

Introduction

> **"Life is extinct on other planets**
> **because their scientists were**
> **more advanced than ours."**
>
> **—Unknown**

If you were born and raised in the United States of America, your vision of how to measure health is certain to be shaped by your past experiences (or not) with doctors and hospitals, by your learned expectations of what it means to get older, by the advertising campaigns of the drug industry, and by the mainstream media in defining all that health should mean to you. Or—if you are among the 20% who swim upstream by exercising regularly and taking the trouble to eat well—kudos to you!

In fact, the concept of health in the American medical mainstream is limited and limiting. It consists of no more than a physical body free of symptoms. In ancient times, in the days of Maimonides and Aesculepius, health meant much more than that. *Mens sana in corpore sano*—a healthy mind in a sound body—implied that body and mind are interactive and that health brightens both sides of that coin. Today, many progressive practitioners work with a new definition of health that includes meaningful work and a sense of spiritual contentment. A purpose in life, a body capable of pursuing that purpose, a calm mind, and a compassionate disposition might define "the life worth living." All life's experiences—benign and otherwise—are lessons. Viewed that way, all the characters that pass through such a life are teachers along the way. This journey and the wisdom gathered from it can then be passed on to others.

> **This planet is a school, and all of its inhabitants are students and teachers both.**

The great deception is that only an expert, a treatment, or a medicine can heal you. The truth is no one knows your body like you do. Though you may go to the "best" doctors, the finest clinics, the greatest healers, no one knows better than you what is happening inside. With improved internal monitoring of physical and emotional states, you can access the healer inside and guide yourself to your answers. The first step to wellness is self-awareness. This will lead to trusting your instincts, which in turn will lead to the greatest journey you could ever take, the self-directed life.

In shifting your "power center" from outside yourself to inside where your inner wisdom resides, you will access the "common sense" which the current system so despises. The term "evidence-based medicine" often makes people feel like they can't know anything, that only the one who has studied for many years can truly understand where to find healing. In fact, your inner healer knows what is best for you. All the scientific studies are no substitute for your personal experience. Remember, nothing works for everyone, and no one knows everything, not even the "best" doctor.

In his simple but powerful book, *The Alchemist*, Paolo Coelho writes, "When you want something, all the universe conspires to help you achieve it." If your goal is the fullness of health, let this book help you put your feet in the right direction, take the first steps, and perhaps awaken to the miraculous opportunity to develop your own power to heal your life. You deserve it, you can do it, and here's how.

> **This book is all about you, your body, its needs, your well-being, and how to achieve it and your ultimate joy in living, which, surprisingly, does not depend on the body or its state of health.**

♪♪♪

You are so much more than your physical body. Just as stepping into a car doesn't make you a Hummer, or a Ferrari, or a VW bus, slipping into a body doesn't mean you are merely physical. The body is the biological vehicle for your soul to experience Earth School. Likewise, this self-regulating, self-healing, intelligent body is more than the sum of chemical reactions or the anatomic arrangement of body parts and is yours to enjoy, revile, abuse, or appreciate. The interplay of spirit and body is what we call life, and a book on self care would be incomplete without a discussion of both aspects of our existence, the finite and the timeless.(Therefore, throughout this book you will find italicized comments that address "the rest of the story," the interface between science and spirituality.) Also, you will find (hopefully) amusing asides, which may be completely irrelevant to the topic. (We take ourselves way too seriously most of the time.) The emerging field of energy medicine addresses the subtle energy "bodies" through interventions that change both the symptoms of illness and the underlying distorted patterns of thought and emotion that generate the symptoms. Energy medicine changes the flow of energy—, - chi, qi, prana-—through the body with various modalities such as acupuncture, homeopathy, Reiki, EFT, quantum healing, therapeutic touch, and many others. (For those who are new to energy medicine, a basic discussion of the energetics of our bodies will be found in Chapter 5.) Physical medicine can be *practiced in perfect harmony with energy medicine, with amazing results. This subject is new to many, but will prove in this century to be an astonishing source of new therapies.*

∫∫∫

Meanwhile, we need to activate and trust our own old-fashioned common sense. It will alert you to ask lots of questions, to seek help inside and outside the medical establishment, and to follow your own instincts to your personal healing. Trust yourself.

"Common sense is all too uncommon."

—Voltaire

∫∫∫

"I am at two with Nature."

—Woody Allen

CHAPTER 1

Conventional Medicine and Holistic Medicine - Know Your Choices

---

"The best six doctors anywhere
And no one can deny it
Are sunshine, water, rest and air,
Exercise and diet.
These six will gladly you attend
If only you are willing.
Your mind they'll ease
Your will they'll mend
And charge you not a shilling."

—Wayne Fields, What the River Knows, 1990

The day I enrolled in medical school, I was filled with excitement. I'd made my choice to become a doctor almost as a mandate from God in my senior year of college. I became possessed with the idea, took two years and fourteen applications before one school took a chance on me. My grades had been mediocre, my MCAT scores excellent, but no one wanted to take a chance on a woman who'd probably quit working as soon as she had her first child. That was the thinking in those days.

But one school did take a chance. The Medical College of

Pennsylvania, which used to be Women's Medical College. Located in Philadelphia, this unique school began taking men for the first time the year I entered. There were 10 men in a class of 100. At holiday time the classroom looked like a sweatshop, with knitting needles and crochet hooks flying as we absorbed neuroanatomy, physiology, and biochemistry lectures.

> **"Get in, get it, and get out" is the surgeon's motto.**
> **So is the even scarier saying,**
> **"See one, do one, teach one." Pithy people, surgeons.**

My first (and only) black bag was given to me the first day of school by a cute little sales rep from Eli Lilly, the drug company. Since it was presented to all of us, complete with stethoscope and otoscope, on the grounds of the school, I thought it was OK—in fact, everything was in right order. We were penniless students who would one day be doctors. This was a sign of the great leap in status we were about to take, through dint of hard work and sacrifice. It seemed fitting that we be regaled and feted in this way by a company which would one day benefit greatly from our power to prescribe. This same sales rep befriended many of us, providing everything from lunches at our student AMA meetings to paying airfare home for a student from California when her mother got sick. It seemed a little strange, but not strange enough to ask questions or object to any of it.

Likewise, the curriculum was not open to question. Since I had decided I was going to be a surgeon, I had very little interest in anything but anatomy. My cadaver was revered, pored over with the kind of rapt attention usually reserved for the dinner menu at a fine restaurant. Biochemistry, physiology—these were subjects for future internists, boring types who would one day take pride in making an esoteric diagnosis or dropping someone's blood pressure ten points. My future would be much more exciting. I saw myself in scrubs, mask, and gloves, up to my elbows in guts and blood, saving lives in the most dramatic way possible. Then I'd happily turn over my patient to someone with more patience to manage electrolytes and the impossibly protracted recovery process. "Get in, get it, and get out" is the surgeon's motto. So is the even scarier saying, "See one, do one, teach one." Pithy people, surgeons.

I practiced ear, nose, and throat surgery for ten years. They'd managed to talk me out of trauma surgery as being basically incompatible with my (guilt-generated) desire to have children. This surgical subspecialty appealed to my pride in my fine motor skills. Much of it is done through a microscope. It requires a steady hand and a sharp eye. Few emergencies arise in the middle of the night, but they do happen. I remember vividly one call at 3 AM to come to the ER immediately to intubate a child with airway obstruction. My two-year-old son woke at that very moment and began screaming when he saw me throwing on my clothes and preparing to dash out the door. It proved way too hard to wake his father, whose involvement with his offspring took place mostly during banker's hours. My sense of panic and despair reached insane proportions that night, and the enormity of my conflicted life came crashing down on top of me. (By the way, I did manage to wake his father, and I did manage to intubate the child who might otherwise have died in the ER that night.) No doctors have an easy life.

After ten years of doing tonsillectomies and ear tube placements, with the occasional thyroid or sinus operation, I decided this was too boring to do for the rest of my life. As luck would have it, the surgical group we had formed—my husband's dream, which I fully supported—fell apart in the malpractice crisis of 1988-89 in Florida. I saw an opportunity and got a job in a (very) small hospital emergency room in central Florida.

ER medicine was exciting and challenging, especially in a small community hospital where there was virtually no back up. I was it! My surgical skills were extremely helpful in situations such as the time they brought in a (female) tractor mechanic whose arm had just been ripped out of its socket, or the occasional auto accident or Saturday night knife and gun club incident. However, the heart attacks and overdoses, the diabetic comas, and the hypertensive crises made me feel inadequate. I began devouring medical texts and reviewing the basic sciences of my early years of medical school.

In the meantime I began meditating on a daily basis, and continued the habit of daily exercise I'd started as a surgical resident in the Bronx. Recognizing how much these two activities were doing for my own health, I wondered why they hadn't even been mentioned in medical school. I began to read about herbs and vitamins. Soon I was giving people lists of things to buy at the health food store, with an admonition to "try this first," as I handed them the "required" prescriptions. I did guided meditations with them to bring down people's blood pressure. At that time (late '80s to mid '90s) I was considered an oddball, an anomaly. One episode comes to mind to illustrate how far I'd come from the "standard of care" and how it was working for the patients and for me.

♪♪♪♪

This is a true story about a life and death emergency that helped start my climb out of the black bag.

I was working a 24-hour shift in a small community hospital in Central Florida, where I often had time to sleep at night. It was one of those quiet nights and I was deep in dreamland, when a loud pounding brought me back to reality very quickly. As my feet hit the cold floor, I slipped on my hospital shoes, wondering what drama would soon confront me. A flood of blinding fluorescent light invaded the room as I peeked into the hall, where a chaotic scene was taking place.

The ambulance doors had flung open to admit two panting paramedics, rushing a stretcher into my ER, nurses running alongside taking the history as they raced the stretcher into the trauma room, where anyone really sick was taken. It was the best-equipped room in the small hospital's ER. As I chased the group down the hall, I heard the sickening sound that told me what we were dealing with. The person on the stretcher was emitting the high-pitched continuous wheeze that is called "stridor," signaling the airway is so tight that the patient can neither inhale nor exhale. This person was having an acute, persistent asthma attack that is called "status asthmaticus" and is fatal in one out of four cases. We were in trouble.

As we entered the trauma room, I could see the figure on the stretcher. A woman's face, ashen, with blue highlights, surrounded by wild blonde hair, stared straight ahead. An oxygen mask was clamped across her nose and mouth by one big hand of a worried young paramedic, who squeezed the Ambu bag with the other. The patient's efforts at breathing were not being effective. An oxygen saturation meter was clamped to her finger and registered a pathetic 78% out of a possible 100. We need 90% saturation or better to function normally. As the medics lifted the patient over to the hospital bed, nurses began opening tubes and locking laryngoscope tongue retractors into place so that I could proceed to intubate the patient, placing a large plastic tube through her larynx and into the trachea. This would provide us with access to her airway until her bronchial tubes could relax and quit squeezing her breath off.

For some reason, the look on her face made me pause. I stared deep into her wide eyes and realized, this woman is not in her body. She is so frightened that she's actually vacated the premises and is floating around out there, terrified!

Her little white feet stuck out from under the thin sheet right in front of me. Instinctively, I grasped the two icicles in my hands and began to talk to her in as normal a voice as I could muster. Shocked, everyone stopped what they were doing and turned to look at me. I was supposed to be in action now, retracting her tongue, visualizing the vocal cords, and gently inserting the breathing tube between them into the trachea below. Instead, I was chatting with her as if this were Sunday afternoon tea and I the Dalai Lama.

"What's her name?" I asked the group, never breaking eye contact. "How are you doing, Diane?" I crooned, trying to make my voice as normal as possible. "What happened tonight? Not your best night, I guess! Don't worry, we'll take good care of you."

She stared straight ahead, but I could see she was coming back, just a little. I kept up the mindless patter, holding her little cold feet at the same time. Everyone was waiting for me to "do the right thing" and put in an endotracheal tube, stabilize her, and send her to the Intensive Care Unit so we could all get some rest.

Meanwhile, someone pointed at the monitor. Our lady's oxygen saturation had gone from 78%, a number incapable of supporting brain function, to 80%, then 82, 84, 89, and hit 92% in less than two minutes. She no longer needed to be intubated. This was unprecedented! No one knew what to do. They started putting away the intubation equipment, sending sidelong glances at each other which mutely stated, "This isn't supposed to happen."

> **That night I had accomplished three things. I'd kept this lady off a ventilator. I'd impressed the staff with something they would learn to call "woo-woo" medicine. And I'd earned forever the nickname "the Witch Doctor.**

))))

The differences between conventional and holistic medicine may be summarized in the following way:

- **Holistic medicine seeks to do no harm**, using gentle methods whenever possible, starting with the least toxic treatments and giving the body time to assimilate them.
- **Conventional medicine shines at acute care**—life-threatening situations where a person's life hangs in the balance and seconds matter. Take me to the ER for a heart attack or a motor vehicle accident.
- **Holistic doctors take time with their patients**, asking questions about all aspects of the patient's life, establishing a relationship.
- In holistic medicine, it is recognized that the beliefs and life habits of the patient are extremely important, and that education into a new way of thinking and behaving is at

least as important as anything the doctor does. As a result, **the doctor becomes a partner in the patient's healing**, rather than the great white-coated expert that must be obeyed. Many patients risk being called "noncompliant" and dismissed from a conventional practice if they don't take the meds—which may be disagreeing with them—or if they refuse to undergo painful and risky procedures.

> *The tunnel vision of conventional specialists—cardiologists, gastroenterologists, and all the other "ologists"—reminds me of the story of the blind men and the elephant. No one sees the whole picture, no one can communicate with anyone else, and the patient is left with utter confusion and too many medications.*

- **There's more than one way to do it** in holistic medicine, whereas the conventional "Standard of Care" defines the treatment plan for everyone, no matter their age, sex, size, or biochemical uniqueness. It's "one size fits all" medicine, and it doesn't.

- Holistic medicine looks for **underlying causes** of symptoms and seeks to correct them. There are reasons why people get sick that go beyond genetics or aging. Exposure to toxins across the years, nutritional deficiencies, infections, unresolved trauma, allergies, and a few other issues constitute correctable, underlying causes in most cases. Symptoms go away when their causes are addressed. Conventional medicine identifies what is "wrong" with the patient, then effectively tattoos that diagnosis (just a label) onto the patient. According to the Standard of Care, there is only one right way to treat a patient. Often the doctor insists the patient must take drugs for the rest of their life. Don't take "sweeping it under the drug" medicines for more than a few weeks. Look for the underlying cause and fix it.

- The **costs** of holistic care are generally far less than the costs of conventional care. For the price of one heart bypass operation (on the order of $100k), twenty people could receive a full preventative course of chelation therapy. The cost of one month of compounded bioidentical progesterone might be $20-30, whereas the same medicine produced by a drug company costs several hundred! The patient doesn't see the costs if they have insurance, but they pay for it in higher premiums.

- Many holistic treatments are **not yet covered by insurance**. So-called health insurance is really catastrophe insurance, just like your car insurance. It pays when you have a problem; it doesn't pay to keep you safe and healthy. If you needed new tires you wouldn't expect Allstate to cover the costs. Does that mean you wouldn't buy tires when you need them? Wouldn't you rather have a choice than be guided by a clerk for where to buy tires or how you wish to be treated medically?

> ***If you needed new tires, you wouldn't expect Allstate to cover the costs.***

As we rocket further into the twenty-first century, we have many choices to make. Not the least is how we structure our health care system. Right now we have an illness care system that makes the disease the enemy, the doctor the hero, and the patient the battlefield. We would be better served by a patient-friendly system of care that covers prevention and stops relying exclusively on high tech (and very expensive) rescue medicine. Right now 80% of our massive health expenditures are spent in the last two years of life! We could include education throughout the school years aimed at teaching kids the proper care and maintenance of their bodies. We could put some effort into upgrading the quality of our food supply, encouraging physical activity, the enjoyment of simple pleasures, and the benefits of communing with the natural world. It would mean weaning ourselves from patent medicines, cleaning up our air, water, food and—perhaps most importantly—respecting the innate wisdom of the body itself. That would seem to be simple common sense, wouldn't it?

> **We currently have an illness care system that makes the disease the enemy, the doctor the hero, and the patient the battlefield...**

CHAPTER 2

The Foundation of Good Health - The Digestive System

Now that the stage has been set, we can look at the nitty-gritty mechanics of the physical body with a holistic eye. We can better appreciate the body's immense intelligence and capacity for healing. Instead of feeling helpless, we grow in our ability to maintain our physical body in great shape through our own efforts. The rest of the book will tackle particular systems. Read the following chapters in any order. Skip the technical parts if you like. Others might find too few of the technicalities. If so, references for further reading are included at the end of each chapter. Look for the pearls that are there for you, incorporate what you are ready for, learn as much as you can, then come back for more. Your journey is unique and wonderful. Remember, life is a learning experience. It's not as important where you start, but how far you go and with what attitude. The world is waiting for your awakening!

Bob was a dance instructor, a tall, elegant man in his early forties. His career as a dancer had been pulled up short because of a debilitating, embarrassing illness called IBS—"irritable bowel syndrome." He'd seen many doctors, specialists in this problem, who'd done all kinds of procedures on him—colonoscopies, upper

endoscopies, X-rays, blood tests, etc., repeatedly for twelve years. He was taking suppressive medication that barely controlled his episodes of explosive diarrhea, and they were beginning to talk surgery. At that point Bob came to see me, hoping for a new approach. He was at his wit's end and was quite depressed about it.

We did a "functional" stool test, which showed us everything about his digestion from mouth to anus. The best part of this test is the microbiology, which, through commonly used culture techniques, identifies the major classes of microbes—bacteria and fungi (yeasts) that populate the intestinal lining.

On the basis of this test, we were able to identify the organisms that were causing this so-called IBS. When treated with the correct antibiotics and antifungal agents, and replacing the good bacteria that belong in the gut, Bob's problem miraculously resolved within two weeks! Since then (ten years ago) he's come back twice for a "tune-up," but he has remained essentially well since that time. He no longer requires any medications, and owns a dance studio where he can practice his great love of dancing all the time without fear of interruption!

PORTAL OF ENTRY

In building health, we do best to begin with the digestive tract. This is our inner interface with the outside world. Just as the skin forms a semi-permeable barrier that defines inside from outside, the gut does a similar function within the enclosure of the body. Not everything that goes into your mouth will be absorbed into the bloodstream. And that's a good thing. In a well-functioning intestinal tract, bacteria, viruses, fungi, parasites and chemical toxins will be systematically destroyed or prevented access to the all-important bloodstream. Let's take a tour of the digestive tract, so we can better understand how to help it maintain our biochemical health.

The digestive tract is really a long tube, which encloses the materials of the outside world within the body. It is an interface with that outside world. Emotional issues impact the functioning of this system in predictable ways. A child with inadequate nurturing will have security/survival-related emotional problems and is very likely to have lower intestinal problems such as constipation, diarrhea, or inflammation of the colon and rectum. Sometimes these problems may come from unresolved issues prior to birth and will occur even in the best of circumstances. It's almost as if the child did not wish to absorb the world as it is. Proper digestive functioning may not occur until the child has been coaxed and cuddled into a more trusting attitude towards life. The root cause of the dysfunction needs to be corrected, through emotional healing with a medical intuitive or energy interventions like acupuncture or Emotional Freedom Technique (EFT).

SENSORY INPUT

Beginning with input from the eyes and the nose, our brain processes information about incoming food before it even hits the mouth. Taste and smell are two senses that help us to select foods that are good for us, and to reject spoiled or toxic materials. The tongue is designed to detect four tastes in various combinations—sweet, salty, bitter, and astringent (think persimmons). If the tongue is accustomed to strong tastes—chemical flavor enhancers, overly sweet or salty foods, etc.—its ability to detect subtler nutrients may be severely limited. Many good food choices may then be rejected, and the wide variety of nutrients that our body requires may not be acquired. In the long run, our health suffers.

Incoming odors and the sight or even the thought of food are enough to begin the process of digestion. Smell is capable of identifying thousands of different molecules in extremely low concentration. Taste depends on a functional sense of smell. Mineral deficiencies may cause a lack of taste and smell. **Zinc** is particularly important for these two senses. This nutritional mineral is found in the outer husk of the whole grain (as are the equally important B-complex vitamins) that is removed when white flour and white rice are produced. These depleted foods are nothing but starch, having had the nutritious minerals and fiber in the outer hull removed. (Food manufacturers then sprinkle a few meager vitamins on the depleted product and call it "enriched." Don't be fooled.) Zinc deficiency can also cause skin problems such as slow wound healing and may be indicated by white spots in the nail beds.

SWEET JUICES

Remember Pavlov and his famous dogs? He'd ring a bell just before food was presented to the canines. Pretty soon, the ringing of the bell was enough to start them salivating, even when there was no food present. Just so with us. The very idea of food, the sight of it, and certainly the smell of it, triggers the saliva glands to release juices into the mouth, which have chemical constituents highly active in initiating digestion. These chemicals are called **enzymes**. The function of an enzyme throughout the digestive tract is to break down food components into smaller and smaller particles, which then can be absorbed through the lining of the intestine. Each enzyme works on a specific type of food. The salivary enzymes work on carbohydrates and are called salivary amylases. They chop complex strings of sugars (starches and polysaccharides) into smaller and smaller pieces (mono- and disaccharides) perfect for the rapid restoration of blood sugar levels. Chewing food thoroughly allows the salivary juices and enzymes to mix well with the food and start the digestive process in the mouth. If your food choices are good, these sugars will be released slowly to keep blood sugar levels stable. If, however, you tend to favor foods high in smaller carbohydrates to begin with, such as those found in sweet drinks, candy, or fruits, blood sugar levels will rise rapidly, then fall just as fast. The yoyo effect this has on energy levels can be very damaging and may over time lead to an inability to properly handle sugars, known as type II diabetes. Choosing longer chain carbohydrates found in vegetables (such as sweet potatoes, carrots, and other root veggies) will feed the body slowly and evenly for hours. The GLYCEMIC INDEX (see www.officialdiabetesblog.com) is a chart of which foods are good starches and which should be avoided. It is also helpful to combine protein and a small amount of the right fats to assure proper nutrition to all the cells of the body. Charts can also be found in *The South Beach Diet* by Arthur Agatston, MD and *The Zone Diet* by Barry Sears, Ph.D.

LIFE IN THE ORIFICE

Many things that happen in the mouth have profound effects on the body. For example, the organisms that live in the crevasses between taste buds, in pockets between gum and tooth, and in the plaque around the base of the teeth will be constantly released and swallowed down the esophagus to the stomach. If they are harmless beneficial bacteria, they will do no damage. However, the simple sugar diet just described tends to encourage the overgrowth of yeast known as Candida species, the same yeast used to bake bread and puff pastries. You can see it on the tongue as a white coating or a sore, red, slick tongue with white spots (called thrush). Further down the line in the gut, this yeast will do what yeast does best—ferment simple carbs into alcohol and alcohol breakdown products called aldehydes. The amount of gas this process produces will cause bloating and great discomfort. The alcohol and aldehydes will cause a constant feeling of fatigue, headache, sinus congestion, muscle aches and brain fog, similar to a hangover.

If for any reason antibiotics are given, further yeast overgrowth will occur. Antibiotics kill off good bacteria that normally take up space in the lower intestinal tract, where they help us digest food. By killing them off, the space resulting will be happily filled by yeast, which is resistant to regular antibiotics. For this reason, any time antibiotics must be prescribed, it is very important to replenish the population of good bacteria, known as **"probiotics."** This is something you can do even though your doctor may forget to remind you, since probiotics are readily purchased at any health food store. **Yogurt, buttermilk,** and

kefir are fermented milk products which contain probiotics, and are a nutritious source of good bacteria. However, they do not provide a concentrated enough source even when used on a regular basis after antibiotics have been in use. To replace large numbers of probiotics, look for a high potency liquid or capsulated supplement that contains both the **Lactobacillus** ("milk bacteria") family, of which "acidophilus" is the star, and the **Bifidobacter**, or Bifidum family. These bacteria help us in many ways, including producing certain vitamins, limiting bad bacteria and yeast, and digesting insoluble fiber in our diet. A healthy digestive tract is home to between 2-4 pounds of good bacteria!

ENERGETICS AND TEETH

Tooth decay and root abscesses are another source of sabotage for the rest of the digestive tract. In addition to seeding the downstream GI tract with bad bacteria, dental problems also influence the energetics of the body. **Baking soda, hydrogen peroxide mouthwash, chlorophyll** in capsules or chewing gum, and **oil of oregano** applied to gums will help keep bacteria and yeast in check. **Coenzyme Q10** is very helpful in healing gum disease. It restores energy to these rapidly replaced tissues.

> *All acupuncture meridians run through the mouth, connecting the teeth energetically with internal organs. Therefore distant problems with heart, liver, and kidney may not be solved unless the health of the mouth is improved.*

BAG OF ACID

Chewing food thoroughly allows mixing of saliva with food, initiates carbohydrate breakdown, and gives the stomach a chance to prepare a welcoming bath of hydrochloric acid and the stomach enzyme, pepsin, for the incoming food. Pepsin is an enzyme that breaks down protein. It works best in an acid environment. Aging can decrease acid production in the stomach. Without it, food will sit in the stomach for a long time, waiting for the signal of lowered pH to move it along. Eventually that food will start to back up into the esophagus, which is not designed for an acid load, and heartburn will be the result. If the stomach's work is hampered by acid-blocking drugs used for long periods of time, like Prevacid, Nexium, Protonix, and Zantac, protein, vitamin, and mineral deficiencies can occur over time. Some associated symptoms might include fatigue, skin rashes (vitiligo, rosacea, psoriasis), bloating and gas, anemia, dizzyness, muscle and bone weakness, tremors, hair loss, and many others.

For individuals whose production of stomach acid and enzymes may be compromised, a supplement of **betaine hydrochloride (or TMG—trimethylglycine) and pepsin** (or other digestive enzymes) taken just before or during a meal, may alleviate the problem of reflux and assist normal digestion to take place.

YEAST AND OTHER BAD BUGS

Another possible cause of "heartburn" is a yeast infection of the esophagus. Yeast overgrowth is fueled by high sugar and starch intake. Soda, white bread, cookies, candies, and cakes all feed yeast. Look at the tongue! A heavily coated white or yellow tongue indicates a yeast overgrowth condition. Careful mouth hygiene, including tongue scraping, must be done. Candida-fighting herbs (**Caprylic acid, garlic, oil of oregano**) or prescription medications such as Nystatin in liquid form or Mycelex lozenges may be used to treat this type of infection. Rinsing with **hydrogen peroxide** or **baking soda** will help kill yeast. **Probiotic** organisms in liquid or capsule form are needed, sometimes for months, to reestablish proper bacterial balance. Of course, of prime importance is eliminating simple sugars and starches in favor of a more healthful, vegetable-based diet. It can take weeks or months to get a fungus problem under control. Constant vigilance is required to keep it from resurfacing, especially if antibiotic treatment or corticosteroids must be given for some other reason.

Our stomach is designed to sterilize incoming material with acid as the food passes through the GI tract. Low stomach acid will allow many organisms, including viruses, fungi, parasites, and bacteria, to get through to the intestine, causing local and systemic symptoms in many cases. Recurrent episodes of diarrhea, bloating, and pain are often the result. Back pain and joint pains are caused by certain toxin-producing bacteria. Acid in the right place is a good thing! Don't make war on your own digestive tract. Heartburn is a symptom of something that needs attention. Taking acid blockers is like taping over the oil light on the dashboard of your car, instead of looking under the hood to see what is going wrong.

ULCERS

In many cases, the lining of the stomach has lost its protective coating of mucus, and the cells of the stomach wall begin to digest themselves, resulting in inflammation and ulceration. Chronic stress can do this. Pain between meals is a good indicator that this is going on. Supplements like **licorice root** (not to be used in individuals with high blood pressure or potassium deficiencies) and **mastic** can help heal this problem. In advanced cases, the ulcer bacteria H. pylori has set up shop and needs to be treated. Usually **mastic gum** (a resin of the mastic plant, not a chew candy) will take care of it, but in some cases antibiotics are required.

B12 AND STOMACH FUNCTION

A healthy stomach is a muscular sac which rolls and mixes the chewed food (bolus) with acid and pepsin and also produces something called "intrinsic factor," a molecule whose job it is to make vitamin B12 absorbable. Of all the B vitamins, this one is the most difficult for the human body to absorb. It is found only in animal source foods, so vegetarians must supplement to stay healthy. In addition to needing a carrier protein called intrinsic factor—which is made in the stomach—B12 from food is only absorbed in the last 9 inches of small intestine! With more than 21 linear feet of bowel and thousands of square inches of absorptive surface, it is only here in the last few inches before the large intestine that this incredibly important nutrient can be absorbed. Any increase in speed of food passage through this area, surgical removal of part or all of it, or decrease in the hair-like surface projections, will severely impact B12 absorption. This vitamin is necessary for normal neurologic function and the production of red blood cells. Lack of this critical nutrient may result in generalized fatigue and neuropathy, that is, numbness and tingling of the lower legs and feet, sometimes also the hands. As deficiencies of B12 worsen, tremors, balance problems, and ultimately death may result.

Vitamin B12 should be given as a sublingual (under the tongue), drop, tablet, or as an injection. It is safe for everyone. Overdoses have never been reported.

INTO THE GUT

When the pH of the food bolus is low enough (acidic), this signals the pyloric valve to open, allowing the food to progress to the first part of the small intestine, the duodenum. Here, digestive juices originating in the pancreas neutralize the acidity. This gland secretes sodium bicarbonate and enzymes such as pancreatic amylase and lipase to further digest carbohydrate and fat. Mixing with pancreatic juice is bile, secreted by the liver and stored in the gall bladder. This bitter, greenish-yellow fluid serves to make fat absorbable. When a fatty meal is deposited in the duodenum, the gall bladder contracts, squeezing its liquid contents into the common duct where the bile mixes with pancreatic juices. From there it flows into the duodenum to mix with the food bolus. Fat is surrounded by bile molecules, which make it water soluble. It can then be carried in the watery plasma of the blood once absorbed. Someone who lacks a gall bladder may have fat absorption problems and should reduce their intake of fat at any one meal. When fat is not properly absorbed, it can be seen floating in the toilet bowl as a greasy scum after a bowel movement. Blockage of the bile duct can cause light yellow or putty-colored stool, since it is bile that gives the characteristic brown color to normal stool. It is also unreleased bile that gives a yellow color to the skin in a person with liver disease.

One enzyme lacking in humans is cellulase, which in herbivore animals like horses and elephants breaks down the fibrous peel of grasses and even the bark of woody plants. It is not abnormal in humans to see corn kernel shells or tomato rinds "exit" the day after a meal of these foods. Beets are notorious for making the toilet water a deep magenta red, which can easily be mistaken for blood. The urine may be similarly colored, but should get lighter quickly over the course of eight to twelve hours. Observing when these things make their appearance can tell you the "transit time" of your intestinal tract. This may vary from only a few hours (too fast) to as much as three or four days (too slow). Normal transit time should be 12-36 hours.

IMMUNE FUNCTION IN THE GUT

> **90% of the body's immune system is found lining the intestinal tract.**

As digestion proceeds, the food moves along the small intestine, where millions of tiny hair-like projections, called villi, absorb the small molecules that provide nutrition to the entire body. *The immune system, our personal Homeland Security, deals with questions of self and not self. 90% of the body's immune system is found lining the intestinal tract.* This is not surprising, since so many would-be invaders try to gain entry here. A healthy intestinal lining is porous only to small-sized nutrients. If the gut lining is inflamed, however, as with heavy metal ingestion, infection with "bad" bacteria, or through eating foods that promote inflammation—like conventionally raised red meat—large particles may leak into the blood. The immune system becomes activated. If larger food particles are mistaken for invaders, food allergies will be the result. Even live organisms like bacteria, viruses, and fungi may sneak through the normally tight area between the cells into the bloodstream.

Allergic problems may start early in life. If the immature digestive tract of an infant is presented foods other than human breast milk, such as cow's milk or soy milk, food allergies will occur in about 4% of children.[1] (This is probably a gross underestimate, since most doctors do not test for IgG-mediated food allergies. The overall incidence of all allergies is 10% of children, including hay fever and skin allergies—IgE type.) Allergies may show up as ear infections or swelling of the adenoids and tonsils, as well as joint pain, headaches, and mood and cognitive disorders. The proper food for a human infant is human breast milk, with just the right proteins, fats, antibodies, and micronutrients, ideally for the first year at least. Other foods may be introduced after six to nine months, but to do so much earlier might be asking for trouble.

The most common food allergens in my practice are milk and other dairy products, wheat proteins (gluten and gliaden), and egg whites and yolks. Egg white is also called albumin and is virtually identical to the albumin protein in human serum. This correspondence can lead to autoimmune disease, where the immune system begins to attack the protein of the body's own tissues. Some autoimmune diseases are thyroiditis (Hashimoto's Disease), lupus erythematosis, scleroderma, vasculitis, etc. All of these diseases originate from disordered intestinal function, which must be addressed and corrected before healing can take place.

Healing a leaky gut may take more than avoidance of allergens. Some helpful supplements are **glutamine**, an amino acid used as fuel by the cells lining the gut, **butyrate**, a fatty acid produced by normal intestinal bacteria, and **"predigested" protein** (some very good fish preparations are available), which will help to heal

---

1   See CDC data at http://205.207.175.93/HDI/TableViewer/tableView.aspx?ReportId=59

and rebuild a damaged intestinal lining. Also, it is never a mistake to push the **probiotics**; they can't hurt you. Herbs can be helpful, including **aloe**, **licorice root**, and **ginger**. In someone with a tendency to develop food allergies, they can become allergic to the herbs. It is smart to take a two-week break every three months, or to rotate herbs. **Flavenoids** like **rutin, quercitin**, and **hesperidin** help cells stick together and prevent leaky gut.

DOWN THE TUBES

In a healthy intestine, yards of tubular small intestine move the liquid food bolus with rhythmic contractions. Nutrients are liberated through mechanical rolling and crushing plus the digestive action of enzymes. Absorption takes place through the villi into the bloodstream. Hormones and neurotransmitters assist the process. In fact, 80% of the serotonin in the body exists in the intestinal tract, and is essential for proper digestion (and you thought serotonin was just there to make you happy?). The entire job of digestion and absorption must take place in the space of a few hours. The corn you eat tonight should be in the toilet bowl the next day. Otherwise intestinal bacteria and yeast begin to ferment the food and putrefaction takes place, producing noxious gas, toxic chemicals, and colicky pain. Without the coordinated functioning of all the components—choice of foods, proper chewing and adequate saliva, swallowing, acid and enzyme production, bile and pancreatic fluids, healthy peristalsis, etc.—the digestive process becomes a menace to health.

Downstream, after transiting the small intestine, the remaining food bolus has become depleted of nutrients. What's left is mostly water and indigestible fiber, along with bile and waste products of metabolism. Turning the corner into the colon, all that remains to be absorbed is water. This water can be loaded with toxins. If it stays too long in the large intestine, it can carry many harmful substances into the blood. This is one reason why constipation is bad for the body. If the waste products remain in contact with the bowel wall for too long, inflammation can set in, which may lead to colitis and precancerous changes in the cellular structure. Constipation, along with the existence of bad bacteria and yeast in the gut, is a very common problem leading to multiple symptoms elsewhere in the body. Think about it! If toxicity is coming from the digestive system itself, where can you hide?

> **If the sewer is stopped up,**
> **the whole house stinks.**

If nutrients are not being provided because of poor food choices and poor digestion, where will the raw materials of a healthy body come from? Poor nutrition cannot be corrected by taking drugs.

Action Points:

- Nutritious food choices
- Healthy teeth and good oral hygiene
- Support of gastric function
- Enzyme and pH support
- Normal evacuation (daily bowel movements)
- Lots of friendly bacteria
- Supportive supplemental nutrients

RECOMMENDED READING:

Optimal Wellness. Ralph Golan, MD, Ballentine Books, 1995. A very readable book about the ten underlying causes of chronic illness.

The South Beach Diet. Arthur Agatston, MD, St. Martin's Press, 2003. Sustainable way to eat, satisfying and healthy for most people. Contains the glycemic index.

The Zone Diet. Barry Sears, PhD, and William Lawren, HarperCollins,

NY. 1995. Another groundbreaking book on the best way to eat for good health and weight control. Glycemic index can be found here.

Why Doesn't My Doctor Know This?: Conquering Irritable Bowel Syndrome, Inflammatory Bowel Disease, Crohn's Disease and Colitis. David Dahlman, DC, Morgan James Publishing, 2008. Begin to heal yourself with this accessible book by a former sufferer.

CHAPTER **3**

What Should I Eat, Doctor?

"No illness that can be treated with diet should be treated any other way."

—Maimonides

ﮞﮞﮞ

"The most dangerous food is wedding cake."

—American proverb

There is so much conflicting information out there in books, in cyberspace, even amongst friends in conversation, it's no wonder most people are confused about what to eat. Let's take a look at the basics of nutrition that seem to work for (most) everyone.

1. **Eat whole foods** – The complete package, as nature presents it, is always better for us than food that has been processed. For example, whole grains contain fiber, important for scrubbing the intestinal lining, and for supporting the growth of good bacteria. The husk of the grain harbors most of the minerals, in particular zinc, an element that takes part in over ninety

reactions in the body. Zinc is important for wound healing, prostate health, and your sense of well-being. Another mineral, cadmium, concentrated in the starchy part of the grain, is toxic because it competes with zinc. So by removing the outer husk, we are getting all of the cadmium and none of the protective zinc. Similarly, whole fruits and vegetables, with their fiber and pulp, slow down the rapid absorption of naturally occurring sugar, sparing the body the trouble of packaging the excess for storage in fat cells. High fructose corn syrup has all the sugar and none of the beneficial components.

2. **Eat fresh, organic, locally grown whenever possible** – Fresh means picked that day or maybe yesterday. Organic means the food hasn't been waxed or irradiated. No pesticides or other chemicals have been used in its cultivation—organic fertilizer only. This clean and naturally produced food contains many more nourishing vitamins and minerals than conventionally grown food. The soil in an organic garden holds moisture and minerals in a buffered state so the plant can absorb what it needs at the time that it needs it. Here, soil bacteria can grow in just the right balance and acid buildup doesn't harm the roots. A depleted soil (no humus, no clay, no soil microbes) provides little nutrition to the plant, so growth totally depends on water and chemical fertilizers. One taste will tell the difference!

3. **Drink plenty of water and few or no sugary drinks** – if there were one habit of Americans that I could change, it would be the consumption of huge amounts of sweetened chemical soup called sodas. I believe these drinks, even (and maybe especially) "diet" drinks, do more to ruin people's health than anything else they put in their mouths.[2]

2   The diet sweeteners all have problems, some more than others. Aspartame (the blue stuff) is the sweetener in most diet sodas. It is a potent known neurotoxin. Don't ever use it. Read labels. Protect the brain cells you have.

Splenda seems to be better. It belongs to a class of chemicals called organochlorides, some of which are very toxic. Sucralose (the active ingredient), however, does not break down and is not fat soluble, so it doesn't build up in the body Stand by for more research. (see http://en.wikipedia.org/wiki/sucralose).

Soda contains water, an important nutrient, but it also contains many other substances in solution that make it harder for the body to extract the pure water it needs. Some of these substances are sugars that attack the pancreas, the adrenals, and the immune system. Some are hydrogen atoms that cause soda (especially cola drinks) to be extremely acid, enough to dissolve a tooth left overnight in a glass of cola. This acidic condition must be corrected in order for many of the body's enzyme systems to work properly. They depend on a constant, slightly alkaline pH (7.4 is ideal) in the blood. The body's buffering (acid neutralizing) agent is calcium, which must be extracted from bones and teeth to balance the acid in the blood. Think of your poor bones dissolving a tiny bit every time you drink a soda! They are!

Water carries waste materials from inside the cell to outside the body. It plumps up the discs between the vertebrae, providing cushion to the spine. It carries nutrients across membranes and comprises 70%-90% of body weight.

Both distilled water and reverse osmosis water have had toxic metals removed, but they've also had the nutrient minerals removed. It is a good idea, especially in hot climates or for people who sweat a lot, to replace electrolytes (sodium, potassium, magnesium, calcium) with a few drops of trace minerals purchased from a health food store, added to a bottle of water. The refreshing properties of a sports drink like Gatorade depends on these minerals. The trouble with sports drinks is the large amount of sugar they often contain to make them palatable to a generation accustomed to super sweet flavoring. In fact, the average American consumes his weight in sugar each year! At one time, refined sugar was a delicacy available only to the very wealthy. (Is that why Henry the Eighth was so portly?)

For those addicted to soda, a good transitional step is to make your own fizzy drinks from fruit juice and club soda. Reduce the amount of juice over time, later transitioning to plain water and decreasing the amount of fruit juice until water in its natural state tastes

Saccharine (the pink packet stuff) has been around since 1907. In the 1960s, a study was done on rats that linked the sweetener to bladder cancer. Since then numerous studies have been done, with conflicting results. No definitive connection has been proven in humans. Still, Canada has declared saccharine illegal, while the US allows its use.

good to you again.

Caffeine is a substance that causes release of cortisol from the adrenals. This is why it energizes, but also why, over time, it can exhaust your reserves. It is moderately addictive. For someone addicted to caffeine, it is best to wean slowly from cola drinks or coffee by substituting water (or herbal tea) for one or two drinks a day, then gradually decreasing the amount of soda and increasing the water. Over about two weeks, done correctly, you will not have to suffer the severe headaches that abrupt caffeine withdrawal will cause.

4. **Eat enough protein for your needs** – Protein provides structure to the body. It is the primary component of muscle cells. It is needed to carry substances in the blood—oxygen, nutrients, hormones—and to keep water inside the circulatory system. It carries messages all over the body in the form of mood-changing neurotransmitters. Protein can be used as fuel when carbs and fats are not available. Enzymes, which catalyze chemical reactions all over the body, are proteins.

How much protein is enough? The experts disagree. Some say you only need one gram for every kilogram of body weight. That means about two and a half ounces a day (at 30 grams per ounce) for a 150-pound person. Half a small burger, a cup of beans, a chicken leg, one egg. That amount can be met with a vegetarian diet, since plants contain some protein too. Others think the body requires more, maybe much more. The truth is that each of us has different needs, and these needs change throughout a lifetime. Certainly needs go up significantly in pregnancy, in times of recovery from injury, or at periods of growth spurts. Protein requirements may also, as Peter D'Amato argues, depend on your blood type. Type O people have been around since the time we were hunter-gatherers, eating whatever we could pick, gather, or kill. Type O's seem to do well on an omnivorous diet, low in grains and high in protein. A and B blood types (RH factor has nothing to do with this) developed after the advent of agriculture, and so are well adapted to a diet of grains, fruits, and veggies. There are exceptions, to be sure, but I have found this to be broadly true, and often counsel patients according to this model. Signs of too little protein in the diet are nails and hair that grow slowly and break easily. Energy is low and the person is often depressed, anxious, or apathetic. Muscles are thin, making the person look angular.

5. **Eat the right fats** – Certain fats are essential for proper functioning of the body and brain. Fats consist of carbon chains with hydrogen atoms attached to some or all of the carbons. They provide the most concentrated source of calories, 9 per gram, of any food source (carbs and protein each provide 4 calories per gram). But they also fulfill other important (structural) roles.[3]

---

3   Why fats are super important:

There are fifty trillion cells in your body (maybe more). Each of them is wrapped in the thinnest of bubbles, only two molecules thick, 13 nanometers. A hundred cell membranes stacked one on top of the other would make up the width of a human hair. One of these molecules (called phospholipids) looks like an old-fashioned paper match which has been split up the middle. A phosphate group forms the water-soluble "head" of the molecule. Dangling from this end are two long (18 carbon) fat segments, like the two "legs" of the match. The fat-soluble legs aim inward in the membrane towards the legs of another phospholipid, forming a chemically stable arrangement. Because oil and water don't mix, one of the phosphate heads projects happily into the watery fluid that bathes the outside of the cell, the other towards the interior of the cell, which is also a water medium. The fats arrange themselves comfortably in between. To prevent drift, long cholesterol molecules insert themselves through the fatty portion of the membrane like mechanical braces, giving it more stability. Large protein complexes form pores, or channels, in the membrane through which substances may enter or exit, according to the needs of the cell inside. The two fatty legs of the phospholipid molecules are precisely arranged. One of them is straight, like the supporting leg of a ballerina doing a pirouette. The other is bent somewhere along its length. Omega nines are bent at the ankle, omega sixes at the knee, and omega three fats are bent at the hip. The molecules spin freely in place. In this way the distances between molecules are exactly determined. The whole membrane is dancing and shimmering, while the protein channels open and close, allowing calcium in, magnesium out, or sodium and potassium likewise to change places, depolarizing the cell. This electrical activity causes contraction or relaxation in a muscle cell, nerve signal transmission in a brain cell, and the wave of electrical activity that causes the heart to beat. Other "receptor" proteins accept and respond to a messenger molecule, such as a neurotransmitter (serotonin, epinephrine, etc.) or a hormone (testosterone, estrogen, insulin, etc.) by changing shape or initiating some new activity inside the cell.

A healthy balance of omega 3, 6, and 9 fats is critical for health. Some of these necessary fats cannot be produced in the body and must be ingested. They are called "essential" fats and are found in **fish oil**, **krill**, and certain plants like **algae**, **flax**, **borage**, and **hemp**. When beef cattle are allowed to eat grass, they too have abundant omega 3 oils in their meat, but most cattle these days are grain fed and no longer have these fats. Instead they have inflammatory ones like arachadonic acid (an omega 6 fat).

When the normal, healthy fats are not abundantly available to form a cell membrane, whatever is coming in through the mouth must be utilized. In this way damaged, deformed, or inappropriate fats, such as trans fats, will be incorporated, causing the membrane to become stiff or otherwise damaged and unresponsive to stimuli from the environment, including hormones. This may be the explanation of such conditions as insulin resistance, adult onset diabetes, metabolic syndrome, lowered immune function, etc. Aging occurs more rapidly when the correct mix of the right fats is missing from the diet.

6. **Eat a variety of different foods** – When people eat the same foods day after day, year after year, they run a big risk of becoming allergic to those foods. The immune system becomes sensitized in certain individuals, especially when inflammation is present in the gut. Also, the nutrients available from those foods are limited, causing relative nutritional deficiencies. Eating all kinds of foods, being adventurous in trying new things, and rotating one's favorite foods, is simply healthier than a monotonous sameness. An innovative diet can also be an exercise in mental flexibility. I always think, "If someone in the world likes this food, maybe I will too!" There are few things I won't try, most of them in the many-legged family of critters. Lobsters excepted, of course!

7. **THIS PROCESS IS AN EVOLUTION, NOT A REVOLUTION.** – Be gentle with yourself, but introduce the needed changes as quickly as you are comfortable doing. Make note of

changes in your body, the way it feels as well as the way it looks. Track the feeling back to the source. Ask your body, not just your mouth, what it likes. Listen!

RECOMMENDED FURTHER READING:

Diet and Nutrition: A Holistic Approach. Rudolph Ballentine, MD, the Himalayan Institute, Honesdale, PA, 1978. Brilliant book about food and its importance in health.

Staying Healthy with Nutrition. Elson M. Haas, MD, Celestial Arts, Berkeley, CA, 1992. Encyclopedic reference book, easy to read.

Optimal Nutrition, Optimal Health. Thomas Levy, MD. This nutrition book is closest to my own philosophy. It stresses the importance of protein in the diet.

Conscious Eating. Gabriel Cousins, MD, North Atlantic Books, Berkeley, CA, 2000. Dr. Cousins' approach is comprehensive and holistic. His philosophy of 80% live food (vegetarian, of course) is hard for many people, but promises to result in bliss and spiritual upliftment. The book is full of good information and is easy to read.

Eat Right for Your Type. The Individualized Diet Solution to Staying Healthy, Living Longer and Achieving Your Ideal Weight. Peter D'Adamo, MD, with Catherine Whitney. GP Putnam's Sons, 1996. If you don't know your blood type, you can donate a pint of blood and they'll tell you. This book makes sense and seems to work for most people.

CHAPTER **4**

What Vitamins Should I Take, Doctor?

**"If I had known I was going to live this long
I would have taken better care of myself."**

—George Burns

There seems to be no health topic more fascinating to the public than this question of which vitamins to take and how much. It is also somewhat controversial, as conflicting scientific studies are trumpeted by the media. This chapter will not answer your questions directly, but will hopefully allow you to make better choices for yourself.

It is tempting for people to try to substitute vitamins for the medications they so fervently wish to discontinue. In the category of "vitamins" they lump many things, including minerals, herbs, homeopathic remedies, and even Grandma's chicken soup! Many people drink cranberry juice to treat urinary tract infections, vitamin C in massive quantities for colds, gallons of antioxidant juices for cancer, etc.

I am not against using any or all of these remedies (they all work to some extent), but it is a mistake to use the simplistic "Take this for that" formula. It simply substitutes nutritional supplements for drugs, and this misses the point of holistic treatment.

> *It is a mistake to use the simplistic "Take this for that" formula. It simply substitutes nutritional supplements for drugs, and this misses the point of holistic treatment.*

We require about ninety nutrients to perform our physiologic functions every day. If we had to know what they do, the daily proportions required of each, and when and where we can obtain these nutrients, we would go crazy and either starve to death or wind up eating everything in sight. Luckily, the body is smarter than the brain in this regard. It has some built-in vitamin-seeking mechanisms that, in the natural state, lead us to healthy choices.

One of these mechanisms is taste. If a food tastes good, it should be good for us. Unfortunately, taste is easily misled. Constant exposure to sweeter-than-sugar sweeteners, extra salty "taste enhancers," and chemical additives of all kinds, has made our tongues numb to all but the most strident flavors. Our children would rather have a greasy iced donut than a juicy peach or a piece of ripe watermelon. They like fire hot salty chips that give them a day's ration of sodium in three bites. No homemade stew, however lovingly made, can compete for our kid's affection with macaroni and cheese from a box, or the ubiquitous carbs-and-fat pizza.

Most of our nutrition should come from the food we eat, and if the diet is abysmal, taking even the best vitamins will not reverse a trend towards poor health. And if the diet is really good, many would argue, do you really need vitamins?

> *Are you old enough to remember the taste—and the smell—of a ripe tomato?*

We can't really know the vitamin and mineral content of any food we eat. So many foods are picked before they are ripe, gassed, stockpiled, and shipped long distances to our stores. Chemical fertilizers can grow pretty fruits and veggies that have little to offer nutritionally. Trace elements are missing from much of the soil in our farmland. (One clue to this is the fact that much of the food has lost its taste. Are you old enough to remember the taste and the smell of a fully ripe tomato?) So to me, the best strategy is to take a "good" multivitamin every day, as a sort of health insurance policy. This assures that at least a little bit of balance gets into the diet. But—be very clear on this—no vitamin supplement can make up for a nutrient-poor diet or a diet full of chemical additives.

So which vitamins should you take? The answer is more complex than we would like. It must take into account the individual chemistry and genetics of each individual. Anyone can pick up a book and read the same recommendations, whether you are a ninety-pound healthy grandma or a three-hundred-pound linebacker with diabetes. It's helpful to know your own body and recognize its responses to various nutritional strategies in order to decide for yourself if something is good for you or not. For example, vitamin C is a great immune booster. Many people take large amounts to stave off colds or to treat the flu. One person might get bowel irritation from one thousand milligrams, another not until three times that much. That's why I've chosen to tackle the vitamin issue in a different way. I'll discuss the different vitamins and you can decide how to use them, if at all.

Our nutritional needs are many. Imagine your body as a symphony orchestra making the music of metabolism. When you tune an orchestra, you don't tune two or three instruments only, because the rest of the (untuned) instruments will bring down the quality of the performance. You can't be sure of the quality of your food, so taking a balanced multivitamin seems the height of common sense, and the best kind of health insurance. It helps tune the whole band of instruments.

The conventional medical literature does publish articles about vitamins. It seems that every year there's a new "glamour vitamin." That lasts until another article is published showing something negative about it, at which point the media pounces and declares that vitamin at best useless, at worse harmful. I've seen that happen with vitamin E, vitamin K, vitamin A, etc. And yet people who take vitamins look better, remain functional longer, and in many cases live longer than their counterparts who don't take vitamin supplements on a regular basis.

Which brings me to the topic of the alleged toxicity of vitamin therapy. In the last twenty years, as many as ten people have reportedly died of a reaction to vitamins. In one year, 2006, the highly respected *Journal of the American Medical Association* (JAMA) reported that deaths from *properly administered medications* among *hospitalized patients only* numbered 106,000! That's the population of Clearwater, Florida, the equivalent of 318 jumbo jets crashing and killing all aboard, or more than twice the number of Americans that died in the Vietnam War! And yet medications are rarely questioned, while vitamins scare people. Go figure!

Vitamin A is found in orange and yellow vegetables, most notably carrots and sweet potato, but not corn. It is good for surface tissues—skin, mucus membranes, and eyes. Without it we have lowered resistance to infections of all kinds. It helps with wound healing and restoring lubrication to dry skin. It is famous for helping with night vision. Because it is fat soluble it builds up in the body, being stored in the liver. (Water soluble vitamins, like C, are not stored.) It shouldn't be taken in excess, but you'd have to eat wolves' livers every day for six months to come up with an overdose, as did an Arctic explorer some years ago. There are water-soluble compounds in these vegetables called carotenoids, which will be turned into vitamin A in the body as needed. Water-soluble vitamins are easily eliminated and cannot cause overdose. A good multivitamin should contain about 10,000 mg vitamin A and maybe 15,000 mg of mixed carotenoids.

B vitamins comprise a "family" of nutrients, since they are often found together in foods, especially the hull of grains (discarded or fed to animals when grains are "refined"), and in Brewer's yeast. Back in 1912, the first of the B vitamins was isolated from rice polish and found to cure the disease called beriberi. These vitamins are critical for nervous system function and for the production of energy. They are important in moving metabolic wastes out of the body. Take them as a **B complex**, since they work together. **Vitamin B12** should be taken in a sublingual form, under the tongue, as discussed previously.

Vitamin C works to support the immune system, acts as an antioxidant, and builds collagen, the protein that holds up the tissues of the body, including the skin structures. It takes four enzymes to make vitamin C in the body. Human beings have three of these enzymes, but not the fourth. All animals except man, primates, guinea pigs, and a few fish species have all four, which is why your dog doesn't need to drink his orange juice every day.

Sources of vitamin C include citrus fruits, melons (cantaloupe especially), potatoes, and peppers.

The RDA (recommended dietary allowance—what I call ridiculous dietary advice) is designed to keep your teeth from falling out, not to achieve optimal health. I recommend a **thousand milligrams** of vitamin C every day. You'd have to eat twelve big oranges to get that much, so taking it in powder or capsule form is much easier. Don't take calcium ascorbate, since it may unbalance your calcium-magnesium ratio and predispose to kidney stones. Any other form is OK, such as **magnesium ascorbate**, **ascorbic acid**, or **ester-C**, a buffered form, which is less likely to cause heartburn.

Vitamin D regulates calcium balance in the body, together with parathyroid hormone. It therefore has a role to play in maintaining bone strength. It is important for mental well-being. The condition "Seasonal Affective Disorder" (SAD) in northern climes has been shown to respond to vitamin D supplementation. It is preventative for serious internal cancers, heart disease, and many other conditions.

We make vitamin D in the skin in response to sunlight. It is therefore important to get out in the sun for 15 to 20 minutes on sunny days (you will make between 8-10,000 IU in that short time), in a tank top or bathing suit. The more skin you show, the more vitamin D you'll make. Of course, don't stay in the sun long enough to burn, since that will increase your chances of developing skin cancer. But remember, we evolved on this planet, that star is our sun, and we metabolize light. So knowing your limits is a good thing, and enjoying some warming rays in a healthy dose is good for you. Common sense works here. If you can't do that or if there is no sunshine where you live, take from **2000-5000 IU** per day of vitamin D3. Ask your doctor to test your "25 hydroxy vitamin D" levels to see that you register 50 or higher. It's much tougher than we once thought to become toxic from vitamin D.

Recent studies have shown **vitamin E** to be protective from heart attacks, perhaps because of its anticoagulant properties. Extra E (beyond that found in foods like nuts and seeds) may be harmful in people who smoke cigarettes (we need more studies to clarify this); however, it has clear benefits for smart people who don't smoke. This vitamin is a powerful protector of the cell membrane, through its antioxidant properties. It also recycles vitamin C. Recommended dosage between **200-400mg** a day. Smokers should take the lower dose.

Vitamin K is important in helping coagulation of the blood and building bone. If you eat green leafy veggies you won't have a deficiency, since only a tiny amount is needed every day. Still, many people are deficient. If you are on blood thinners such as Coumadin/Warfarin, your doctor may tell you to stay away from greens. That is an ignorant attitude. Salad is good for you and rat poison (Coumadin) may not be. Keep eating salad and let your doctor adjust your dose.

MINERALS

Minerals are elements that take part in almost every chemical reaction in the body. We've already seen how they may be depleted in the soil. Organic produce is grown without chemical fertilizers and is much more mineral rich than conventionally grown produce. Ground-up rock (especially granite) is a great fertilizer to use in your garden, since it contains all the minerals. So is fish emulsion—smells nasty but grows excellent plants.

- Balance is key with minerals. **Calcium** must work with **magnesium, sodium** with **potassium** and **copper** with **zinc.** So many people, especially women, are taking large amounts of calcium in an effort to keep their bones strong, but no one has ever told them to take magnesium too. The result of taking unbalanced calcium is progressively worsening insomnia, anxiety or depression, muscle twitches, and heart rhythm disturbances. All these may easily be corrected with equal doses of calcium and magnesium (taken in divided doses, magnesium supplements won't cause diarrhea). Magnesium is absorbed through the skin also, so a warm body bath or foot bath with Epsom salts (magnesium sulfate) is a great way to relax and harmonize your system.

Since the amount of minerals in the body depends on the amount you take in, plus your ability to absorb them, you can get a hair analysis to see the sum total of your mineral status. A good laboratory to use is Trace Elements in Arlington, Texas. Many health practitioners use this test, though few are medical doctors. It is helpful to see a nutritionist, a nutritionally oriented doctor or chiropractor if you've got chronic health issues, or as a preventative strategy.

Take home points:

- Take a good multivitamin most days. "Good" means it has high enough dosages to make a difference, especially if you are new to taking vitamins or have been taking the usual M&M size shellac-covered multivitamin most people take. Your body's needs are not met by these RDA doses.
- Two 1000mg capsules of fish oil (EPA/DHA) daily wards off an astounding number of ailments, including chronic pain. Flax oil may be used but is not quite as beneficial as the fish stuff.

- Do testing to see what you really need, as opposed to trying every new "miracle" that comes along.
- In the same spirit, educate yourself about specific medical conditions your parents or you may have and which nutrients have been shown to be helpful in these conditions. Look for actual science, not just claims by the people who stand to profit. You will be amazed at how many studies have been done, and also how many more need to be done in order to bring nutritional treatments into the mainstream.
- Work with a professional who is qualified in nutrition. This is especially important if you have a chronic or undiagnosed "medical" condition. No condition falls out of the sky. There is always a reason for it, even though your doctor may not know what it is. There is a doctor somewhere who does know. Ask at your local health food store, look on the Internet, and never quit seeking what you need.

For **further information**, I recommend the following websites:

www.orthomolecular.org/library/articles/index – excellent library of scientific studies in nutritional treatments of chronic illness. Worth a browse. Physicians will find these articles are rigorous and educational.

www.pubmed.gov – the National Institutes of Health website of published data archived from the scientific, peer-reviewed literature. Huge, daunting database, sometimes hard to find just what you want to see, but probably the largest source of primary scientific literature on the Web.

RECOMMENDED READING:

Diet and Nutrition. Rudolph Ballentine, MD. Delightfully written, not at all boring as the title might lead you to believe.

Encyclopedia of Nutritional Supplements. Michael Murray, ND. Exhaustive list of supplements, what they do, how to use them, written by a naturopathic doctor.

Textbook of Functional Medicine. From the Institute of Functional Medicine in Gig Harbor, Washington. For the technically minded. Physicians beware, this information may rock your world.

CHAPTER **5**

The Anatomy of the Energy Body

One of the greatest disappointments of my medical education was the complete lack of philosophical discussion. When you're learning to deal with human suffering, birth, death, and all the vulnerabilities that patients bring to the medical encounter, it would help to have deep probing talks with experienced professors, to read and discuss Chekhov and Maimonedes. Philosophical discussions were never part of the program. Instead we were taught by example to stuff our questions and our feelings, to leave the poetry to poets, to handle things in a detached and stoic, "scientific" way. We came to believe that death is our eternal enemy, that we are never to question why— only how—to keep someone alive. We have no guidelines to help us answer the question of when is it OK to let someone go. We learn how to talk to the family without showing any feelings of our own. This gives doctors a cold and aloof appearance that is the antithesis of compassion.

The closest we get to a spiritual practice in medicine is the ritual of scrubbing for surgery, a cleansing ceremony without a heart. We cut people open without reverence, without prayer, without humility, without compassion. The soul of medicine has been stuffed into an old file cabinet and locked away amongst the dusty books of herbal lore and the tattered remnants of the alchemist's cloak. Anything not "scientifically validated" is despised and dismissed, including the patient's own observations of what is going on in her body. In our drive to be detached and scientific, we have systematically forgotten why we do what we do.

> **The soul of medicine has been stuffed**
> **into an old file cabinet**
> **and locked away amongst the dusty books of herbal lore**
> **and the tattered remnants of the alchemist's cloak.**

Still, in odd moments, at the bedside of a dying old man, perhaps, those ancient issues come into focus. Watching the process of dying unfold—the feathering of the breath, the draining of color and life force as the person slowly detaches from his body—can induce feelings of reverence for life. Mystery has always been a part of life that science does not comprehend or appreciate. Death is sometimes an enemy to be fought with every tool you have; at other times it is a welcome ally that brings peace and closure to a long struggle.

It is helpful to look at the mind-body connection through the model of the yogic or the Chinese medicine tradition, where energy has been recognized and respected for thousands of years. The shamanic worldview (the medicine of all indigenous cultures around the world) places the individual within the community of all living things—Nature, cosmos, the wheel of life. To connect these ancient insights with modern scientific tools makes any clinician much more powerful.

〜〜〜

In both the Indian and the Chinese systems, it is recognized that there is an energy flow in the living body. This flow is circular, like an electric current in a circuit, and interacts with energy flows around it. It is strong or weak depending on many factors, and determines the person's state of health. Any impediment to the natural flow weakens the body and creates pockets of dysfunction, which manifest as sensations of discomfort or pain. The location of the dysfunction is a clue to the underlying pathology, which always has its origin in the energy body, not in the physical. Even accidental injuries can be seen as disruptions of energy first, since the "victim" is often distracted by a mental thought or an emotional issue before the accident, causing or allowing it to happen. Sometimes an accidental injury occurs when that person is in dire need of a rest period. She might be unwilling to create that "time out" for herself due to perceived life demands and pressures. Often the body will manifest an injury to get that needed rest.

In yoga philosophy, the life energy flows from the ground upwards, from Earth to Heaven if you will, passing through the human body as if through a transformer. We feed from the physical—food, water, air, sunlight—and transform those physical substances into thoughts and emotions, creations of the human spirit.

THE CHAKRA SYSTEM

As the energy flows upwards, it encounters seven centers of increased activity, vortexes that concentrate energy, called the chakras. These are not anatomic structures and cannot be found in dissection or on an X-ray. They can be sensed with the hands, with the "vision" of an intuitive person, or with sensitive electronic equipment. These seven centers download energy to internal glands and organs, which interface with the body by producing the hormones and neurotransmitters that regulate internal physical processes. Let's look at how this works in detail.

FIRST CHAKRA – SECURITY, TRUST

The first chakra is located at the base of the spine. It is pure potential and must unfold its way upwards as growth and development occur. This is the center that activates at birth and develops throughout childhood. Its nurturing emotion is a sense of security. The child learns that this is a safe and loving universe through the consistent and caring actions of nurturing caregivers, usually the parents and family members. A strong emotional bond feeds that sense of self within a loving community, and the child has a healthy emotional foundation on which to grow in consciousness toward the light. If instead a child is abused or neglected early in life, damage occurs in the first chakra. This injury may result in a deep insecurity or a feeling of intense shame. This is a difficult—but not impossible—obstacle to overcome later. The associated parts of the physical body are the skeletal system (the underlying structure) and all the surfaces where interactions take place between the individual and the environment. These include the skin and the immune system, as well as the inside of the digestive tract where food, germs, and toxins are ingested and absorbed or rejected.

SECOND CHAKRA – PUBERTY

About the age of 12 or 13, the second chakra becomes activated. This new energy produces characteristic changes in the body and the mind that we call puberty. The voice deepens, secondary sexual characteristics develop, new interests come alive, and childhood toys are set aside. A new and profound change has occurred. The sex glands mediate these changes through their production of hormones.

A healthy second chakra balances the male and female parts of the self. The yin/yang symbol is the perfect representation of a healthy second chakra, - black and white, male and female, - the marriage of opposites.

Unhealthy development here may result in pelvic pain, disturbed hormone balance, sexual maladjustments and distorted self image.

Being the generative center, the second chakra is the source of raw creative power.

THIRD CHAKRA – POWER IN THE WORLD

The third chakra opens and blossoms in young adulthood. Its theme is the acquisition of power. This is the ability to make one's way in life, to take care of oneself financially, professionally, and as an individual developing his personal power in a practical sense. He finds his niche through testing himself competitively, getting an education, learning to pay bills, care for a home, find a partner, get a job. A person with a healthy third chakra will be self-confident, self-assured, calm, and centered. The chakra is located in the geographic center of balance of the body, the "solar plexus"—the "hara" of the martial arts. Related organs are the stomach, the liver, the spleen, the kidneys, and the pancreas. Too much energy in this center will result in arrogance and domineering tendencies, stored anger (liver disease), gastritis, heartburn, gall bladder problems. These people are often competitive and hard-driving and may be extremely successful in their work. Too little energy here results in low self-esteem and lack of confidence in self. It also appears as a false bravado that is used to cover up deeper feelings of inadequacy—a "macho" kind of swagger that is common in young men who are seeking to exact from others the "respect" they haven't yet earned for themselves. Ulcers and kidney problems occur from fear and anxiety that are the emotions that accompany low third chakra energy.

> *Love is the elixir that shifts one from a self-centered worldview to a broad based spiritual understanding of life.*

FOURTH CHAKRA – LOVE

The fourth chakra centers at the heart. It involves the emotions of love, compassion, connection, and gratitude. A healthy heart chakra will both radiate love and accept love that is offered from people and the natural world with openness. Love is the elixir that shifts one from a self-centered worldview to a broad based spiritual understanding of life. Sometimes the heart center is activated by a spiritual experience, such as St. Teresa of Avila's ecstatic experiences in prayer and meditation. More commonly it comes through romantic love, which is seen by the rational mind as nothing less than insanity. Love is an activity of the heart, not the mind, and cannot be understood in a rational framework. This is why people shake their heads at lovers—love looks just like madness.

People with an abundance of third chakra energy often have dammed the upward flow of energy to the heart and have serious problems maintaining relationships, both at work and at home. Because the body is by its nature a poet, working with metaphor and not words, it may produce in these individuals a narrowing of the coronary arteries, symbolic of the heart starved for love. Type A personality people have more "heart attacks" than other, better balanced people. The community in the US that has the lowest rate of heart attacks is composed of close-knit, extended Italian families who live, love, and eat much as they did back in Italy.

Some people have a lot of heart energy, but have developed a habit of giving all that energy to others, producing a lack of self-love and nurturing. This is a personality complex that often goes along with cancer. It is interesting to speculate why the breast, the only organ whose sole function is to donate nourishment to others, is so often the site of cancer. Perhaps a new line of research might be opened into identifying such characters early in life and helping them balance the tendency to give away too much of themselves before they get cancer. It is thought that all disease is 20% genes, 80% environmental factors, even cancer.

In medicine we are quite comfortable and familiar with the energy of the heart as measured by the electrocardiogram, the EKG. It is not so well known, though, that this energy is measurable to a distance of at least 15 feet off the surface of the skin. This means that whenever we are in proximity to one another, our heart fields are busy interacting. Perhaps we are able, on a subliminal level, to sense this energy, and this is why we are drawn to certain people. Their energetic patterns (not just the heart, but the whole system) create synergies or interference patterns with our own. Much research has been done on "resonance" and "entrainment," as these phenomena are called.

The lungs are also located within the fourth chakra sphere of influence. In Chinese medicine, they are considered to be the seat of grief. Indeed, the breath is a good indicator of the state of the emotions, being deep and slow when relaxed, becoming high and shallow under stress. Conscious deep breathing automatically signals the nervous system that all is well and can be used in any situation to help relax the body. Asthma is often related to food allergies or other environmental and emotional triggers. The body's defense system is attacking normally harmless substances in a kind of paranoia that does more harm than good. In a similar way, many people who've experienced pain in love will reject any further opportunities to explore love again. The drawbridge goes up, the gates are closed, and the defending army hurls fiery arrows from the ramparts, pushing away the very thing that offers nourishment to a starving heart.

FIFTH CHAKRA – SELF-EXPRESSION, WILL

The fifth chakra is located at the base of the neck, near the thyroid gland and the larynx. It concerns itself with self-expression. This is where one finds her voice, her will, her mission in life. It is the refined expression of the creative impulse that is generated in the second chakra, the center of generativity. Here it becomes art, music, dance, stories, architecture. This is the first center that is uniquely human. Animals have all the lower ones, including the heart, but no animal can create in the way that we do.

Deficient fifth chakra energy results in feelings of lack, of frustration, of the damming of the natural flow of heart energy upward towards God and the highest impulses of humankind. Everyone has a "song" he came to sing, and the suppression of this song may result in problems with the voice, the thyroid (too low or too high metabolism, goiter, cysts, cancer) or in heart palpitations from abnormal accumulations of energy.

SIXTH CHAKRA – THIRD EYE

The sixth chakra is normally called the "third eye," as it is located above and between the eyebrows, inside the skull. It is your internal TV screen, where intellect and imagination play to the internal audience, your witness, the soul itself. It is also the place where messages are received in an extrasensory way. Sudden flashes of insight, inspiration, channeled information, cosmic downloads are received here. (Intuition is a little different—it is a whole body knowing.) Sixth chakra is the part that's hooked in to the human grid, and perhaps the interdimensional grid as well. Dreams are received here—messages from the collective unconscious, in all their trappings of fantasy and metaphor. The third eye is a power tool for receiving information that may be couched in mystery. It can be a fun place to be or a frightening one. Ignoring or suppressing psychic information can lead to headaches, eye problems (refusing to "see"), and in the worst case, strokes and brain tumors. High functioning of this chakra has led to some of the greatest breakthroughs in all human endeavors. The chemist Kekule worked on the problem of the structure of the glucose molecule for many years. He knew it was six carbon atoms linked together, but he couldn't get how it was constructed until he had a dream of a serpent with its tail in its mouth. Of course, glucose is a ring structure. Accessing the dream world solved the problem.

SEVENTH CHAKRA – DIVINE CONNECTION

The task of a lifetime is to clean up the obstacles to energy flow by learning your life lessons. This allows you to become a clear channel for the transformation of density to light. We, as human beings, must tackle our personal obstacles, which consist of emotional blockages, outdated and negative conditioning, ego defenses and habits, which no longer serve. When we do this, and diligently strive for the highest and best we can be, our upward energy flow meets the constant stream of incoming light from the higher realms, which pour into the seventh chakra all of the time. This meeting of the lower and higher selves causes a nuclear explosion, which is called by the yogis Samadhi, by the Buddhists nirvana.

It is a blissful state where the individual merges with the Universal, all is understood, forgiven, transformed, and dissolved in the overpowering knowledge that all is Love. This is the purpose of the whole game. In the acknowledgement of Oneness, the Cosmic Game of hide and seek is done. The seventh chakra is wide open.

ↄↄↄↄ

The Chinese system is also based on energy flow, depicted on the surface of the body by fourteen meridians—the central meridian in the front midline and governing meridian in the back midline, plus six paired meridians on either side of the body. Each pair relates to an internal organ, which can be influenced through the stimulation of access points along the length of each surface meridian. The internal balance of the body is managed by the dependency of each organ upon the other and the interplay of opposing qualities such as masculine/feminine, Yang/Yin, heat and cold, dry and damp. The whole system is tied in to the hours of the day because each (paired) meridian and its corresponding internal organ is activated for two hours of the twenty-four hour day. For example, an excess of lung energy might mean the person can't sleep between the hours of 2 and 4 AM, when that meridian is activated. A deficiency of spleen/stomach energy might have the person napping every afternoon. In addition to the skilled use of acupuncture and acupressure, balance in the body can also be achieved through the use of warming and cooling herbs. This is the basis of Traditional Chinese Medicine. The ancient martial arts and the healing system of qigong, of which Tai Chi is a part, rely on an understanding of energy flows, interactions, and the use of earth energies by the individual. Stylized and ritualized movements direct and balance the body's energy flow within the electromagnetic energy of the earth itself.

PROCESS OF DYING

The process of dying is the ultimate test of control of conscious awareness. A fully conscious yogi detaches from his body by loosening the energetic body from the physical at each chakra, detaching one at a time, bottom to top, finally exiting from the crown chakra towards the light. A shaman—an indigenous healer—can

> ***A conscious, peaceful death can be a great blessing to the individual and also to his family.***

assist the process by "unwinding" the chakras for the dying person in a specific order. Those in attendance will witness the process, perhaps intoning prayers, chanting, or playing sweet music to allow the soul to leave bathed in peaceful and loving vibrations. Contrast this image with the frantic, painful, often violent efforts to keep the soul in the body that Western medicine inflicts on everyone, like it or not.

There is a time and a place for everything, and a premature death should be opposed by every means possible. However, in certain circumstances even in the Western world, a conscious, peaceful death can be a great blessing to the individual and also to his family. A philosophy that leaves room for dying enhances the quality of life for every individual, since we must all die eventually. The hospice model has gone a long way towards providing death with dignity for many thousands of people.

꩜꩜꩜

A friend of mine was present at the death of her father. He had been ill for a long time, and his passing was appreciated, if not welcomed by the whole family. They sat in attendance as a harpist played gentle music and the old man breathed his last. Several people in the room saw a luminous wisp rise from the bed at the very moment of transition. But all of them saw the lovely butterfly that entered through an open window, fluttering about over the heads of everyone in the room for what seemed a long time before leaving through the same window.

RECOMMENDED FURTHER READING:

The HeartMath Solution: The Institute of HeartMath's Revolutionary Program for Engaging the Power of the Heart's Intelligence. Doc Lew Childre and Howard Martin. HarperCollins, New York, NY, 1999. Based on real scientific research, the HeartMath Institute gives practical steps for achieving better heart (and mind) function.

The Anatomy of the Spirit: The Seven Stages of Power and Healing. Carolyn Myss, PhD, Three Rivers Press, New York, NY, 1996. Dr. Myss presents the chakra system in all its glory in a full-length book.

On Death and Dying. Elisabeth Kubler-Ross. Scribner, New York, NY, 1997. This is the landmark book that woke up a nation.

Sacred Mirrors. Alex Grey, Ken Wilbur, and Carlo McCormick. The visionary art of Alex Grey offers the best images of the human energy field I've ever seen. I call it "The New Gray's Anatomy," as it updates the classic text we learn from in medical school.

CHAPTER 6

The Healthy Heart

"Drop the mind that thinks in prose;
Revive another kind of mind that thinks in poetry.
Put aside all your expertise in syllogism;
Let songs be your way of life.
Move from intellect to intuition,
From the head to the heart,
Because the heart is closer to the mysteries."

—Osho

The heart is that tireless great drum that provides the background rhythm to our lives. First, the mother's heart, pulsing and pounding, the maternal metronome that calls us into life, the beat of which will forever calm us and cradle us. Then our own heart, big as a fist, working and working and working, awake or asleep, young or old, that brackets our existence from the first unto the very last beat.

A healthy heart beats about 60 times a minute. The average (not so well conditioned) person's heart beats about 80 times a minute. Over a lifetime of 80 years that adds up to between 2.5 and 3.36 billion beats! What can you do for your heart, that it may beat steady and strong for many decades? Following are some things you need to know that you probably never learned in school.

ANATOMY AND FUNCTION

Heart function depends on 1) coordinated action of the heart muscle, 2) rhythmic electrical wave propagation, and 3) proper function of four valves (tricuspid, pulmonary on the right, mitral and aortic on the left). Finally 4) muscle strength depends on mineral balance and sufficient proper nutrients to feed the working cells.

The job of the heart is to pump blood around the body. There are four chambers, the right atrium, right ventricle, left atrium, and left ventricle. On the right side, blood from the body, loaded with waste materials and carbon dioxide, is received from the vena cava into the right atrium. From there it drops into the right ventricle and is pumped through the pulmonary artery into the lungs, where the CO_2 is exchanged for oxygen. Back through the left side of the heart, the newly refreshed blood is pushed out the aorta and thence through the arterial side of the circulation to all the corners of the body. Hidden in the root of the aorta as it exits the heart are the openings for the coronary arteries, which nourish the heart muscle itself.

ELECTRICAL ACTIVITY AND RHYTHM

The rhythm of the heartbeat is orchestrated by electrical activity in the heart muscle cells themselves. Each and every cardiac cell is electrically active and can generate a pulse beat on its own, which it will bravely do even if isolated in a petri dish all by itself. However, some cells are more equal than others. The orchestra conductor is the sino-atrial (SA) node, in the right atrium, which initiates the pulse. The electrical charge is then carried down a narrow bundle of cells between the ventricles to the interventricular (IV) node. This intermediate station then splits the signal so it is carried to each of the ventricles separately. The progression of depolarization is perfectly timed to allow the atria to fill, then empty, pushing blood into the ventricles while the big chambers are relaxed. The muscular ventricles then contract and shoot their contents to the lungs and the body in a coordinated wave. One-way valves between the chambers and another pair at the exit holes assist in directing the blood flow properly and preventing backflow.

BLOOD PRESSURE

The pressure generated by the pump directs the blood into the arteries, which are tubes that have muscle tissue in their walls, allowing them to narrow (contract) or dilate (relax). The combination of heart pumping action and arterial back pressure determines the blood pressure. The systolic pressure is the maximum generated at the peak of each ventricular contraction, the diastolic pressure is the low number, representing the "resting" blood pressure at the bottom of the relaxation phase. The amount of blood per beat and the ease of its passage depend on clean arteries and the proper contraction and relaxation of the heart itself. The heart muscle is be nourished by the relatively small coronary arteries—left anterior descending (LAD), circumflex, right coronary artery (RCA), and their even smaller branches.

CARE AND FEEDING OF THE HEART

The heart is the only muscle in the body that never rests. As a result, it has enormous metabolic needs and must itself be fueled adequately. It requires plenty of glucose and oxygen to burn, as well as numerous nutrients, vitamins, and minerals for all the work it must do. One of the important substances required for proper functioning is Coenzyme Q10, found in every cell's mitochondria, the body's energy-generating factories. The more metabolic activity a cell is asked to do, the more mitochondria it will have. It is in the mitochondria that adenosine triphosphate (ATP), the energy molecule itself, is made. The heart has many more mitochondria than any other organ, and a greater need for CoQ10 to produce energy on a continuous basis. It is well known that the statin class of drugs, used extensively to lower cholesterol, works because it blocks the action of the enzyme that produces cholesterol, which is *the same enzyme that generates CoQ10!* Anyone on statin drugs should be counseled to take CoQ10 to protect all their muscles, especially the heart.

HEART DISEASE, OUR NUMBER ONE KILLER

More people in the US die of coronary artery disease (CAD) each year than any other single cause. In fact, more than 300,000 deaths happen annually in people who never had a symptom or sign to indicate that they had a problem! Another 300,000 deaths occur per year in people with known CAD. In 2005, 2,400 people died *per day* of heart attacks. Another 1.3 million that year had a cardiac event that was not fatal.[4] Women are as much at risk as men—this is one unwelcome sign of equality of the sexes. Known risk factors include a family history of heart disease, high cholesterol, elevated markers of inflammation in the system (*C-reactive protein, homocysteine*), smoking, inactivity, and *being unhappy in your work.* Heart disease patients have a particular personality profile too—they tend to be overachievers, hard-driving and hard workers, although they may not like their jobs. More heart attacks happen on Monday morning than any other day of the week. Routine cardiology assessment may fail to uncover a heart problem until the heart attack actually happens. Ask for an assessment of your risk factors beyond the lipid (cholesterol) profile.

Here are the risk factor prevalence for heart disease among adults according to the Center for Disease Control (for years 2003–2004 unless otherwise noted):

- Percentage of persons aged 20 years and older with **hypertension** or taking hypertension medications: 32.1%
- Percentage of persons aged 20 years and older with **high blood cholesterol**: 16.9%

---

4   Heart Disease and Stroke Statistics-2009. Circulation. 2009; 119:e21-e181.

- Percentage of persons aged 20 years and older with physician-diagnosed **diabetes**: 10.0%
- Percentage of persons aged 20 years and older who are **obese**: 32.0%
- Percentage of adults aged 18 years and older who are current **cigarette smokers** (2004-2006): 18.4%
- Percentage of adults aged 18 years and older who engage in **no leisure-time physical activity** (2006): 39.5%[5]

Looks like at least some of the major risk factors are modifiable and don't require drug therapy, namely inactivity, obesity, and cigarette smoking. In a study from the year 2000, the CDC showed that 76% of adults don't smoke, only 40% have a healthy weight, 23% eat 5 or more fruits and vegetables a day, and 22% exercise on a regular basis. The number who do all 4 of these healthy things for themselves is only 3% of the adult population of the United States![6]

CONVENTIONAL TREATMENT

The treatment of heart disease in conventional medicine includes the use of drugs—aspirin, beta-blockers, lipid-lowering drugs, and blood pressure meds like angiotensin-converting enzyme (ACE) inhibitors—and bypass surgery or angioplasty with or without stent placement. These surgeries carry substantial risks. One study published in the journal *Circulation* showed an incidence of 26% adverse events (death, stroke, repeat MI, or need for repeat procedure within one year) in the group receiving stent placement, vs. 12% for bypass operation.[7] A meta-analysis of the results of such surgery showed little difference in overall survival, with both procedures often requiring re-operation within five to ten years. The

---

5   www.cdc.gov/heartdiseasestatistics/htm

6   Circulation. Lloyd-Jones et al. 119(3):e21(2009) http://circ.ahajournals.org/cgi/reprint/CIRCULATIONAHA.108.191261

7   Serruys PW, Unger F, Sousa JE, et. al., for the Arterial Revascularization Therapies Study Group. "Comparison of coronary-artery bypass surgery and stenting for the treatment of multivessel disease." N Engl J Med. 2001; 344:1117ñ24.

underlying process leading to heart disease has not been altered with surgery, but time has been bought during which the individual can change those factors over which he has control.

COMPLEMENTARY THERAPIES YOU CAN DO

It is worthwhile to review the current thinking about what causes coronary artery disease. At first, inflammatory proteins are found in high concentration in the blood. *Where do they come from?* One, homocysteine, is an intermediate by-product of protein metabolism. It shouldn't stay as homocysteine for long, but it cannot move along to the next stage without adequate amounts of vitamin B6, B12 and folic acid. Many people are depleted in B vitamins due to eating processed foods and having poor digestion. This one is easy to fix.

C-reactive protein is a general marker for inflammation. This blood protein will be high if inflammation is present in the system, such as a urinary infection or a sore throat. But it will be persistently elevated in persons who eat a lot of meat. The fats in the meat create an inflammatory substance called arachadonic acid that attacks the lining of the arteries. Wherever blood flow is turbulent, the arterial wall can be damaged by inflammation, leading to an abrasion or ulceration of the normally smooth wall. The body patches this inflamed area with something like a clot. Fibrin threads form a matrix to which platelets then adhere. Cholesterol then gets in the act. Along with calcium it forms an insoluble patch, like plaster on a wall in your house. This patch will continue to grow and harden, leading to narrowing of the artery and gradually choking off blood flow. In a coronary artery, this will lead to poor heart muscle function even before an actual cardiac "event" can happen. The cardiac event usually consists of a clot forming in the already narrowed vessel, or a piece of softer plaque "rupturing" and blocking completely the flow of blood. Within minutes, heart muscle begins to die.

Understanding this process allows for interventions at numerous points to actually prevent the event from taking place. First, inflammation can be kept at a minimum (even in meat eaters) by lavish helpings of fresh, organic vegetables and fruits, loaded with **antioxidants** that quench inflammatory free radicals. Eating fatty fish (salmon, sardines, herring) and taking **fish oils** has been shown unequivocally to decrease inflammation by shunting fats away from the arachadonic acid pathway. For this reason they are also excellent at reducing the pain of arthritis and other inflammatory conditions. Clot formation can be discouraged by taking **blood thinning** vitamin E, plenty of fish oil, and many herbs, including ginko, garlic, ginseng, and ginger. Be careful with these if your doctor has you on blood thinning drugs like Coumadin, aspirin, or Plavix.

Of course, it is well known that a graduated program of **exercise** as well as **avoiding inhaled toxins** (cigarette smoke, one's own or someone else's) are preventative too. Identifying and avoiding food allergens is important and will improve heart health as well as decreasing inflammation in the whole body. Supplemental CoQ10 is mandatory for those on statin drugs. One hundred mg a day is good, 200 mg is better. Cholesterol can be very effectively reduced with oat bran, fish oil, inositol hexaniacinate (a natural form of slow-release niacin), and by optimizing hormone and thyroid function (see Chapter 3). Often cholesterol levels normalize and patients no longer need statin drugs. It should be said that statins have an antioxidant property too, which may be why they can be helpful beyond the capacity to reduce cholesterol levels. Still, this is an expensive and unnatural way to address the underlying problem of inflammation.

ONE POWERFUL AND SAFE THERAPY

A powerful anti-inflammatory treatment that also improves circulation all over the body is **chelation therapy.** One of the most efficient ways chelation can be administered is as an intravenous (IV) drip in the doctor's office. With repeated treatments, chelation slowly removes the hard calcium from plaque, allowing the obstructing plaque to gradually wash away in the blood flow. It removes toxic metals from the body, which both decreases inflammation and unblocks chemical processes by replacing the toxins lead, cadmium, or mercury with the nutrient mineral (zinc, copper, iron, etc.) that belonged there in the first place.

SCIENTIFIC STUDY OF CHELATION THERAPY

The principle objection of the medical community to chelation therapy has been that proper scientific studies have not been done. At the time of this writing there is a large-scale prospective, double blind, placebo controlled study that is designed to prove or disprove the theory that chelation really is a good treatment for this type of heart disease. It's called the TACT trial—the Trial to Assess Chelation Therapy. With a generous grant from the National Institutes of Health, Dr. Gervasio Lamas, chief of cardiology at Miami's Mount Sinai Hospital, is the principle investigator. He is an exceptional practitioner because he listened to his patients. Many of them told him about their experiences with chelation, or asked him questions about the treatment that he couldn't answer. So he decided to undertake this definitive study. The results will be revealed in 2010.

Those of us who have been offering chelation therapy for years know already what it can do. The rest of the medical profession knows little about the process, but is usually quick to condemn it.

About twelve years ago, the father of my son's best friend, a man of about fifty, who had already had bypass surgery once, was told that he needed another operation to open the clogged bypass vessels. He refused, stating he would rather die than face that surgery again. At the time he was unable to walk from his front door to the end of his short driveway without getting winded. His quality of life was poor and he was resigned to whatever would happen. He came to us for help. Sal had about forty chelation treatments over the course of a few months. During that time he became progressively more energetic. He took up an exercise program and took the vitamins we prescribed with diligence. He eventually did so well that he moved back to his beloved New York City and got himself a new life!

Twelve years later he is still going strong, with occasional chelation treatments to maintain his gains.

THE RHYTHM IS GONNA GETCHA

The regularity of our heartbeat is not only reassuring to babies and pets, it allows for the most efficient pumping of blood to occur. As the ventricles are compressing, shooting a fistful of blood into circulation, the atria are at the same time relaxing and filling. The next moment, the empty ventricles are being filled by the squeezing action of the atria. Blood returning to the heart through the vena cava and pulmonary vein backs up until the atrium relaxes and the valves open. It is the coordinated timing of this pumping action upon which proper circulation depends.

Any other type of pumping action will be less efficient, and some very uncoordinated electrical signals in the heart can kill a person in minutes. An irregular rhythm in the atria will cause less blood to enter. In the ventricles, an arrythmia can result in the heart muscle twitching like a bag of worms (fibrillation) with no pumping action at all. A too fast rhythm (tachycardia), even if it is coordinated, doesn't allow time for the chambers to properly fill, and may compromise circulation. Too slow (bradycardia) and not enough blood is pumped for the brain to stay functional.

What is the cause of such life-threatening rhythm disturbances? It may be a congenital abnormality of an electrical pathway. These show up very early in life. More often in adults, rhythm anomalies are due to irritability of the heart muscle because of an imbalance of the minerals and hormones in the blood.

For example, if a woman is taking large amounts of calcium over time, without enough of the balancing mineral magnesium, the muscles all over her body will be more likely to spasm. Calcium is an excitatory mineral, while magnesium relaxes muscles. The rush of these two minerals back and forth across the muscle cell membrane "depolarizes" the cell and causes contraction. When an imbalance affects the heart, independent contraction of heart muscle cells or bundles will disrupt coordinated contraction and lead to an arrythmia.

During the years of menopause and perimenopause, or with prolonged stress in anyone, imbalances and sudden changes in hormone balance can destabilize heart rhythm and cause runs of "palpitations." These are propagated waves in the bloodstream that occur when blood, trying to get into a chamber, slams against a closed valve when that valve should be open. Again, timing is everything.

In these cases, balancing the hormones or the minerals can correct the problem very easily. The longer an arrythmia exists, the tougher it is to correct.

Other causes of arrythmias are too low or too high thyroid function, disturbed coronary artery circulation, heart attack or slow death of dominant pacemaker cells, trauma, lack of sleep, prolonged anxiety, drugs, caffeine, and probably others that we have yet to discover.

Sometimes these imbalances can be corrected by balancing nutrient minerals or hormones. Extra magnesium given intravenous has been shown in the emergency situation to relieve many types of arrythmia. Taking it by mouth is a strategy you can begin at home. Fixing the sleep problem, the hormone problem, or the thyroid problem should be done with competent help. In many cases, anti-arrythmia drugs must be given while these corrections are underway. If you have heart palpitations or blood pressure problems, you should give up caffeinated drinks too.

FEED YOUR HEART

Nutrients which improve cardiac performance are many. Magnesium is one of the most important, as we have seen. The balance of calcium and magnesium is fundamental to proper muscle function. In a balanced individual, the intake of calcium should be twice that of magnesium. In someone who has been taking calcium alone, it is usually necessary to give equal amounts of the two nutrients for some time before balance is achieved. The reservoir of calcium in the body is the bones. This is also true for magnesium. This mineral is essential for more than 300 chemical reactions throughout the body. It is found in all kinds of greens (it's in chlorophyll), grains (quinoa and buckwheat), salmon, and seeds, - pumpkin, sunflower, sesame and mustard. Epsom salts (magnesium sulfate) in a bath can help restore balance too.

Coenzyme Q10 is made in our cells (unless we're on statin drugs), is found in meats, and of course is also available at health food stores as a supplement. It is a fat-soluble nutrient and so should be taken with meals. CoQ10 is essential for generating energy inside the cell's mitochondria.

Carnitine and **taurine** are amino acids that improve heart muscle function. **Ribose** is a fuel that feeds heart muscle preferentially. The herb **hawthorne** causes heart muscle to contract more forcefully. **Human growth hormone** and **testosterone** reverse in many cases the wasting condition called cardiomyopathy, which leads to congestive heart failure.

UNDERSTANDING THE HEART FIELD

The heart generates a huge electromagnetic field which is detectable at least fifteen feet away from the person. Better instrumentation will reveal it to be much larger still. This means our "heart fields" ARE CONNECTED TO EACH OTHER ALL THE TIME. The signature vibration of a heart will resonate and connect with the vibrations of another in a unique way, often causing us to feel instant attraction or instant dislike for that person.

In examining the underlying causes of heart disease, we must include the energy of the fourth chakra. Is it balanced or is it blocked? It is well known that a certain personality type, the hard-driving workaholic, is disproportionately affected by heart attacks. Could this be because the tremendous energy concentrated in the third chakra, the work center, the power center, leaves little upward motion of chi to power the heart? The body is a great poet, so the metaphor of blocked coronary arteries can be interpreted as a heart starved for love and joy, missing the essence of life in a vain attempt to find it in possessions or power in the physical world. Without changing this dynamic, the heart patient cannot truly heal. We repeatedly get ourselves into the same mess, physically and emotionally, until we learn the lesson of that situation and move on to the next problem scenario. This is the nature of Earth School. It is smart to look for the lesson in every situation so that you don't need the proverbial "cosmic 2 by 4" to make you pay attention.

RECOMMENDED READING:

The Heartmath Solution. Doc Childre and Howard Martin. HarperCollins, New York, NY, 1999.

www.heartmath.org The organization doing much of the scientific research on heart-brain coordination and the role of stress in heart disease.

www.cdc.gov/heartdisease/statistics/htm Government statistics on heart disease in this country.

www.americanheart.org American Heart Association website, statistics, suggestions for healthy living. Extensive scientific documentation for conventional interventions is accessible here, but alternative treatments are not even mentioned.

CHAPTER 7

Brain Health - Now and Forever

"Never engage in a battle of wits with an unarmed person."

—Oscar Wilde

The brain is the organ of greatest mystery. It senses the world outside from a distance, interprets information from all parts of the body, governs life processes within the body, and navigates the soul's physical experience from inside its little bony capsule. It is the central processing unit for information pouring in from the fifty trillion cell cooperative community that is the body.

It is also a modest three pounds of soft tissue, 1.8 pounds of which is fat, voraciously utilizing 20% of the body's blood supply, and 20% of the body's glucose. It requires a constant level of oxygen and will die within five minutes deprived of breath. It measures life by the rhythm of the stars, governing the physical body by the rising and falling of the sun and the moon in the sky.

We have only recently begun to understand the complex functioning of this 3-pound wonder. From the 1950s when neurosurgeon Wilder Penfield operated on un-anesthetized persons, awakening vivid past memories by touching parts of their exposed brain, the brain's functions have been elucidated more and more.

New tools of investigation have brought new information and new mysteries to unravel. We still don't understand the chemistry of thought or the biology of sleep. We can image the brain's anatomy with MRI and CAT scans. PET scans allow us to see specific areas of the brain light up as it "does its thing." We can analyze the chemistry of a brain cell. But ask a neuroscientist what makes one person a genius and another a fool, and he will laugh. (What is laughter?) We're not there yet. We've just found out that nerve cells *can* regenerate, but we don't know how to *make* them do that. We know there is electrical activity going on in the brain, but we don't yet see that we might be connected electromagnetically with each other and with the electromagnetic field of the planet itself.

MYSTERIES OF CONSCIOUSNESS

> ***Where is the mind and what is it?***
> ***Is consciousness a by-product of brain chemistry***
> ***or is it the fundamental organizing principle***
> ***of the universe itself?***

Let's look at some of the new science and the intriguing questions it raises.

In the 1970s physicist-researcher Dr. Elmer Green conducted a series of tests, which became famous as "the Copper Wall Experiments." He put practiced meditators in an electromagnetically shielded room with a copper-lined wall that was able to pick up electrical emissions at a distance from the subjects. Sensitive electronic equipment was placed on the other side of the wall. No one could see inside the room and the meditators could not see out. As the meditations got deeper, Dr. Green expected to see subtle fluctuations in the voltage meter. He saw nothing. Over and over again, the experiment was repeated, and to his dismay, nothing registered. It was not until he changed the settings on the detector that he saw that instead of a subtle change in voltage, he was getting shifts a thousand times stronger than what he had expected! The signal was so strong, it had overwhelmed his recording equipment! The power of focused attention was proven to be extreme. What a surprise! (*Is this the brain at work, or the mind? How does one relate to the other? Where is the mind and what is it? Is consciousness a by-product of brain chemistry or is it the fundamental organizing principle of the universe itself?*)

Many advances have come about in the intervening years, and yet we still understand so little. Elmer Green's own wife developed Alzheimer's dementia in her later years. Because Dr. Green, a respected brain scientist, had psychic abilities himself, he was able to "go with" his wife across the mental boundary to whatever dimension her consciousness was now occupying. He was able to understand the dynamics of dementia in a way no one had before. The effort has raised even more questions about the nature of mind and its connection to the physical body. Dr. Green's book about the experience is called *The Book of the Ozawkie: Alzheimer's Disease is Not What You Think It Is*.

In a series of well-designed studies, the Institute of Noetic Sciences, an organization devoted to research in consciousness, demonstrated the interrelatedness of consciousness. A subject was placed in a closed room with video cameras in the corners. As she went about her business, she was wired to monitor blood pressure, pulse, and galvanic skin response. In another part of the building, far from the room, another individual would look at a monitor, which at random times would show a real-time picture of the first subject. The subject's vital signs responded every time she was being watched, even though she didn't know it. The response was more marked when the observed and the observer were of opposite sexes! Repeated testing with many different subjects yielded similar results.

Recognizing that we understand very little about the workings of the brain lets us examine the strategies we can employ to keep our brains as functional as possible, as long as possible.

NUTRITION FOR SMARTS

Brain nutrients range from simple glucose (sugar) to hormones. The bulk of the brain is composed of fat, so if we are to keep it healthy, we can only eat the purest, healthiest fats throughout our lives. (See Chapter 5.) Omega 3 fats are as important to brain function as they are to proper heart function. Quality fish oil should be pharmaceutical grade or molecularly distilled to remove toxins and to avoid a fishy taste that happens when oil goes rancid. Cholesterol is important to make those nerve cell membranes structurally sound. Extra virgin olive oil, grapeseed oil, butter, and coconut oil are preferred to corn oil, soybean oil, or cottonseed oil for cooking. These oils are preferred for their balance of essential oil content and their resistance to heat damage at normal cooking temperatures. That means it's smart to avoid all deep fried foods and anything fried that you might be tempted to eat outside the home. Overheated fats make poor cell membranes. Fish, flax, borage, hemp, and evening primrose oils are all useful to build proper cell membranes in the central nervous system. Control your fats, control your destiny!

Recently a story appeared in our local paper about a female pediatrician whose husband, 53 years old, was showing the earliest signs of Alzheimer's disease. He'd forget not only where he put things, people's names, and what he ate for breakfast, but was losing the ability to find his house. When she realized what was happening, she began a methodical search for nutritional supplements that might help him. What she discovered was that a tablespoon a day of **coconut oil**, either straight up or mixed into a shake, soup, stew, or used as a cooking oil, completely reversed his symptoms. Worth a try in anyone who shows unusual memory loss, or as a preventative treatment for all of us. Coconut oil does not denature at higher cooking temperatures. It does not raise cholesterol.

Mineral balance helps the brain to send electrical transmissions cleanly and crisply down the wires, the neuronal axons, which can be up to three feet long! Balanced sodium and potassium, as well as calcium and magnesium, are the key minerals in nerve transmission. Dietary imbalances of these minerals are common. Much depression, insomnia, agitation, and irritability is due to the practice of taking calcium supplements without the balance of magnesium. Adding magnesium to the diet in the form of greens, or using supplements or soaking in Epsom salt baths, will help to correct that problem. Toxic metals can unbalance and poison the nerves, replacing the nutrient minerals, causing neuropathy, fatigue, pain, and other mischief.

The vitamins vital to brain function are vitamin C and the B vitamin family. Thiamin, B1, is often deficient in alcoholics, among others. These people, when stressed, can experience temporary psychosis or even death as a result of thiamine deficiency. It is common practice in emergency rooms all over the country to give a dose of thiamine to every alcoholic who passes through the doors.

Vitamin B12 is so important, and yet so difficult to absorb, that it deserves special mention. When deprived of B12, anemia results and individuals commonly display fatigue and uncoordinated movement that can progress to shaking, muscle weakness, and inability to walk. The deficiency is much more common than most doctors recognize, and since requirements vary widely between individuals, blood levels can be very misleading. To be safe, take 1000mcg as a sublingual (under the tongue) tablet or liquid several times a week. Since, as nutrition expert Dr. Jonathan Wright puts it, "The only way to overdose on vitamin B12 is to fill a bathtub with it and drown in it!" you should be quite safe in doing so.

ݕݕݕݕ

Recently in my practice, a gentleman was seen who had just been given a diagnosis of amyotrophic lateral sclerosis, or Lou Gehrig's disease—an incurable progressive deadly disease of the nervous system. An astute associate, Dr. Todd Gracen, recognized that the fellow's hair analysis indicated low mineral levels across the board (a sign of poor absorption usually due to inadequate stomach acid). Especially low cobalt (a component of B12) clued the doctor to the likelihood that the patient was B12 deficient. He began giving him injections of B12. To everyone's surprise the patient began to improve rapidly, achieving full normal function within a month of starting weekly injections. He continues to take these injections and is today quite normal.

♪♪♪

Other specific brain nutrients include **Coenzyme Q10** and **alpha lipoic acid**. These fuel, respectively, energy production in the brain and the health of the cell membrane. They turn on gene sequences that clean up the toxic by-products of metabolism. **Acetyl-L-carnitine**, **vinpocetine**, and **ginko biloba** improve blood flow, memory, and nutrient utilization by the brain as well. **Coconut oil** has recently been touted as an effective treatment for the memory loss due to Alzheimer's disease. Studies remain to be done, but meanwhile common sense would dictate that it should be used in cooking. These are only a few of the nutrients that can help restore or preserve normal brain function. **Chelation** therapy helps maintain nervous system health by removing neurotoxins like aluminum, mercury, and lead. (See Chapter 10.) We all have these stored in our bodies to a greater or lesser extent, and are more or less susceptible to dementia depending on our genes and our eating and exercise habits throughout life.

Hormones are an important part of brain health. The clinical picture of dementia—confusion, severe memory loss, atrophy of brain tissue, dehydration of the brain—happens far less often in women who take **estrogen**, since estrogen is supportive of brain function. Some people continue to produce their own hormones to some extent through life, but most women need some hormonal support. Sometimes just the precursor hormones **progesterone** and **pregnenolone**, from which the body can make estrogen, are enough. Men in later years usually need testosterone to maintain normal brain function and mood.

SLEEP, THE GREAT RESTORATIVE

One of the most important factors in healthy brain function is the amount and the quality of sleep you get. Scientists are mystified by sleep—its function, its mechanisms, but there is no doubt that sleep is restorative, and lack of it causes dysfunction to a greater or lesser degree in everyone.

When I was much younger I remember a disc jockey in New York, my hometown, attempting to go without sleep for a week. He was on the air continuously for the whole time, and his speech became progressively less crisp, more garbled, less coherent, until he had what seemed to be a psychotic episode and the experiment was terminated after about five days. I never heard what the long-term effects were on him, but we know that sleep deprivation breaks down normal thinking and is used as an interrogation technique all over the world.

Sleep seems to reset normal brain function. It clears out moods, attitudes, and accumulated aggravations of the day. It's Nature's refresh button. Just for fun, let's speculate on how this might happen.

THE GEOGRAPHY OF DREAMLAND

If we can agree that energetic processes go on all the time in the body, then we can speculate on how energy circulates and interacts with the larger energy fields in which we are embedded. In Chapter 3, we presented in detail the human energy field and some of its important points of contact with the outside world. Now let's look at brain waves in particular, for they have a striking correspondence with resonant frequencies of the Earth itself. As I was beginning to develop this theory, I came across the book The Mayan Code *by Barbara Hand Clow. She writes in detail about this very idea. This is what she proposes.*

Our waking consciousness, our "normal" state, produces brain waves from **13-40 Hz** (Hertz, or cycles per second). This is called the **beta wave** state. The molten iron core of the Earth vibrates at this frequency range. We are resonating with the very heart of the planet during our normal state of functioning.

As we drift into a more relaxed state of mind, but still awake, **alpha waves** are generated at a frequency of **8-13 Hz**. The **Schumann resonance** of the Earth's surface, caused by lightning strikes all over the planet that reverberate through the atmosphere, vibrates at exactly this frequency range. Coincidence?

In a state of light sleep our brains tick along at **4-7 Hz, the theta wave**. This is also the frequency of the outer atmosphere, between the dense inner atmosphere and the innermost Van Allen belts of radiation that circle the globe. The Van Allen belts consist of charged particles that are held in place by the magnetic field of the Earth, the same way that iron filings are drawn to a magnet.

The deepest sleep we experience takes place at a frequency of **1-4 Hz, the delta wave** state. Outside the atmosphere, from the outer Van Allen belts onward into the cosmos, this is the frequency we find.

♪♪♪♪

Why would we have a system that requires us to resonate every night with the outer reaches of the planet and the solar system? Is it possible that we "plug in" at night and literally "recharge our batteries" through resonant connection with the electromagnetic energies of the universe itself? Do we dump our debris in the outer dimensions and come back clean and ready to connect again with the planetary energies the next day? Isn't it a miracle that we are so very attuned energetically with our home planet, and doesn't that make perfect sense? Both the dream state and the dreamless condition of deep sleep are absolutely necessary for normal daily function.

While the consciousness is off in hyperspace, what happens to the body? It goes into a state resembling hibernation. Heart rate and breathing slow down, metabolism goes down to only what is required to maintain essential functions, the body is put on auto pilot, and the spirit takes flight to the outer reaches of who knows where? The rational mind is left behind, having little to offer in the exotic realms of Dreamland.

This intriguing model of what sleep might actually be doing raises questions about the artificial energy fields we have created with our electronic devices. How do these impact our brain function? Do cell phones, with their microwave radiation, cause disruption? What about the electrical activity that is generated in the mouths of millions of people from mixed metals used in dental work? Can this be strong enough to interfere with normal brain activity? How much interference can the brain handle? All these questions must await scientific recognition of the extreme importance of energy in the normal functioning of the human body. Until we can look at the physics of the body as clearly and objectively as we do its chemistry, we can have no answers. But we can find some interesting facts through inner explorations of our own experience. Meditation is the systematic exploration of one's inner experience that gradually changes the experience of the outside world and has been used by every culture throughout time, with the exception, until recently, of ours.

PHYSIOLOGY OF SLEEP

Certain hormones are released more at night. One of them is melatonin, the sleep hormone, which is also a powerful antioxidant system and which responds to the presence or absence of light. Shining a light on the back of the knee (or elsewhere on the skin) will shut down melatonin production! Sleep hygienists say the room you sleep in should be as dark as possible. I think we can get away with a little light, since there have always been stars in the night sky, but the bright light of the full moon may be too much for us to sleep well. Melatonin comes from the pineal gland in the dead center of the skull. It is the metronome, the timekeeper, the master gland that tells the rest of the system when to sleep. Pushing through the sleepy signals at night is a bad idea, since this is the ideal time to go into deep states. Later on, sleep may not take you all the way to the delta wave state, so you are missing part of the night's journey and its restorative properties. This stresses the adrenals and interferes with adrenal recovery.

Through sleep, the adrenal glands are reset. Cortisol production rises, to peak in the morning when all systems must be mobilized again. Cortisol is an energizing hormone. It starts out high in the morning and dwindles as the day wears on, reaching its low point about midnight. The state we call "burnout"—caused by overwork, strong emotions over a long period of time, or lack of rest—is actually accompanied by low adrenal cortisol.

The other nighttime hormone is human growth hormone, which is usually thought of in context of teen growth spurts and acromegalic giants. Actually, growth hormone in the adult has a restorative function and directs tissues to repair themselves. People who supplement growth hormone generally report more energy, tighter skin, better muscle mass, and an overall feeling of well being. As we age we release less and less of it, but it is released mostly at night.

MORE GOOD STUFF FOR THE BRAIN

Proper brain function depends on exercise—physical exercise for the body, and mental exercise for the mind. As we have seen, physical exercise increases blood flow and oxygen-carrying capacity. It releases stored toxins, and it causes endorphin release in the brain.

Exercise for the mind means learning new things, such as studying a language or learning to use a computer. It means exercising our considerable creative ability, perhaps in interior design, cooking, beading, or knitting. Writing, speaking, learning to paint or play a musical instrument, etc., can contribute to longer, better mental functioning.

Reading is an activity that exercises the mind, especially when new information is being absorbed. The moment of realization of a new idea has been called a "brain orgasm" or an "ah-ha moment," and feels immensely rewarding.

Of course, doing puzzles and games are fun and challenging activities. They too can be a part of maintaining brain function. So can continuing work activities and managing one's own affairs. The more an elderly person can remain independent, the better they will function. Being responsible for another being, even a pet, can also encourage better brain function. Older people with pets live longer and report happier lives than those who are completely alone.

So, as with the rest of the body, good brain function depends on proper nutrition, exercise specific to the organ, physical exercise of the body, sufficient high quality sleep, and eliminating toxicity.

RECOMMENDED READING:

Brain Longevity: The Breakthrough Medical Program that Improves Your Mind and Memory. Dharma Singh Khalsa, MD, and Cameron Stauth, 1999.

Magnificent Mind at Any Age: Natural Ways to Unleash Your Brain's Maximum Potential. Daniel G. Amen, MD, 2008.

A Younger You: Unlock the Hidden Power of Your Brain to Look and Feel Fifteen Years Younger. Eric Braverman, MD, McGraw-Hill, 2008.

The Mayan Code: Time Acceleration and Awakening the World Mind. Barbara Hand Clow and Carl Johan Calleman, PhD, 2007.

The Book of the Ozawkie: Alzheimer's Disease is Not What You Think It Is. Elmer Green, PhD.

CHAPTER **8**

Sex Hormones in Women - The Good and the Not-so-good

Before we start, ladies, I want to offer a word to the men who are reading this book. It's not that I'm ignoring you, or that I don't recognize that men experience hormonal issues throughout life, especially when testosterone levels begin to decline in the fifties and beyond. It's just that a man's issues are so simple they don't warrant a whole chapter. The answer is—take testosterone and take care of yourself. Find a practitioner who knows the difference between patent drugs and natural hormones and get tested. If you want to stay young, virile, handsome, and fit all your life, exercise like crazy, eat well, and take your hormones. Don't let your woman do it for you—she can't. If she's looking good and you're not, there may come a time when she just doesn't want to look at you any more. Now on to the complex side of the human equation: women.

WHERE WE'VE BEEN

Before the 1950s, women suffered through menopause with little support from the medical community. Kitchen remedies like herbs, castor oil packs, and ceiling fans were about the best we could do. (I remember a beloved aunt sitting at her kitchen table, red and sweating, fanning herself with her skirt.) Sometimes women were institutionalized for symptoms of mental instability due to menopausal imbalances. In the 1950s we had the introduction of Premarin, and the controversy about hormone replacement has been raging ever since.

Premarin, in case you haven't heard, is made from PREgnant MARe's urINe. Horses are kept in confinement, kept pregnant, and the distillate of their collected urine is fed to women. Is it any wonder it causes problems? Chinese emperors and empresses did the same, only they used the collected urine of their finest (human) athletes. Horse urine contains equine estrogens and estrogen breakdown products, none of which are native to the human body. Whenever unfamiliar (or newly invented, patentable) hormones are introduced into a live human body, unpredictable effects happen. Natural hormones cannot be patented in the USA. Therefore no profit can be made from proving to the FDA that they are safe and effective. No monopoly on sales will be conferred. Therefore no drug company is interested in developing or marketing them. There is no profit in natural, but there is safety and efficacy, way beyond any newly created hormone, or distilled hormone from another mammalian species. These hormones were sold and marketed to American women for decades before adequate testing showed in what ways they were helpful and in what ways they were harmful. The Women's Health Initiative was published in 2002. It was the first large-scale study on the effects of Premarin, funded by the drug company Wyeth-Ayerst, the manufacturers of this type of HRT (hormone replacement therapy). They were certain the results would show definitively that estrogen replacement from horse urine is unequivocally helpful for postmenopausal women. Instead the results were mixed. Breast cancer incidence was increased by nearly 20% in those taking synthetic progestins, while colon cancer incidence was reduced by 15%. Symptoms of hot flashes were relieved, bone density stabilized, but other symptoms were no better.

It seemed that overnight, the entire gynecologic profession reversed their direction. Previously they had stampeded in the direction of putting every woman on hormone replacement. After the publication of the Women's Health Initiative, they suddenly reversed direction and stampeded all their patients away from hormone replacement.

From my vantage point, having used bioidentical (natural) human hormones for years in my practice and on myself, I was confident that I was *doing no harm* to anyone. This new piece of information didn't affect my practice in the least. It simply proved that using invented patent medicines does not have predictable results. Imagine putting long side chains on the basic hormone skeleton, creating synthetic hormones that never existed on this planet, and then giving them to people to see what will happen! Is that what Hippocrates had in mind? I don't think so!

So remember whenever you read about hormone studies in the magazines or newspapers, be sure you know which hormones, or (so-called) "hormones," are being studied. Most likely they are not the natural hormones, since no one will put up the funding for their study as no one stands to make a fortune by selling them.

REAL VS. INVENTED

The three estrogens that are native to the human body are estradiol, estrone, and estriol. The male hormone testosterone differs from estradiol, the principle human estrogen, by *one hydrogen atom*. Look at the world of difference that tiny change produces—greater body size, deep voice, hair everywhere, and a brain so different in men and women that I call it God's practical joke to have put us on the same planet! Now imagine a lab scientist in some dark little corner of a great pharmaceutical company, creating molecules from estradiol that have never existed before, hoping that this one will be the contraceptive or the menopause patentable drug that won't make her nose fall off or her pubic hair grow down to her knees! (Some side effects are just too weird, even women won't put up with them!)

THE DANCE OF THE HORMONES

Here's what happens each month in the female body during her reproductive years. Estradiol does a little dance during the lunar month (the moon rules women, in case you hadn't noticed) that causes one egg among hundreds of thousands to ripen and release, two weeks into the cycle. It thickens the lining of the uterus, plumping it up with a bed of blood vessels in preparation for the implanting of that egg in case it should have a lucky encounter with a team of sperm. (Only one sperm achieves the goal, but all of them are necessary to get him there—ever wonder why men love team sports so much?)

At the moment of sexual climax, millions of sperm are catapulted into the "birth canal" and begin a journey as tough as the Tour de France. They struggle across the boggy uterine lining, bathed in acidic fluids, then swim blindly down the corrugated Fallopian tubes, half of them taking the wrong turn. Deep within the correct tube the ovum awaits, bouncing slightly in her excitement for she knows not what!

It is not the first sperm to find the egg that is the chosen one. In fact—and here is the point—NO SINGLE SPERM CAN ENTER THE EGG until there are thousands of others covering her outer membrane, activating her energetically and chemically, softening her defenses, warming her up, so to speak, for the lucky hero to penetrate the goal, the egg's nucleus, the Holy of Holies.

The rest of the team will all die and be flushed out or eventually absorbed. But what a game it was!

**"I can't believe that out of millions of sperm,
you were the quickest!"**

—Steven Pearl

Immediately after the release of the egg, the ruptured follicle cyst begins to produce the hormone progesterone—the hormone that supports pregnancy. Recently published studies in the gynecologic literature recommend supplementing natural progesterone in women who've had multiple spontaneous miscarriages. (Why not test in advance of these little tragedies, and replace progesterone in women who need it?) Patent progestins don't work for this purpose, or you can bet they would have been recommended first. The drug of choice for this condition back in the '50s was a horror called DES (diethylstilbesterol, an invented steroid hormone). It wasn't until *the daughters of the women who'd taken it* started showing up twenty years later with vaginal cancers that the long-term damage of this particular hormone started to be known. Apparently the misery caused by this one drug is also passed along to the daughters of the daughters, for who knows how many generations, should they live that long!

If implantation of a fertilized egg does not take place, both estradiol and progesterone fall rapidly. The hormonally unsupported uterine lining is allowed to slough, causing menstrual bleeding, and the whole dance begins again.

THE RIGHT BALANCE

Now that is how the dance should go in a healthy, hormonally balanced, nutritionally supported woman. In our culture more women than not have menstrual irregularities, imbalances, and a consequent slew of symptoms due to (usually) too much estrogen and not enough progesterone. Let's look at the different effects of these two classes of hormones so we can understand where the symptoms come from, and the right way to relieve them.

Estrogen is given to cattle to fatten them up for market. Progesterone, on the other hand, has activity similar to male hormone (testosterone). It is classified as a weak androgen and occurs in men as well as women. Progesterone slims the body and balances the unopposed weight gain caused by estrogen. When progesterone is lacking—either because it is not being produced, or because it is robbed by overactive adrenal glands to make the stress hormone cortisol—premenstrual syndrome (PMS) occurs. The few days right before the period become quite uncomfortable. Breast soreness occurs due to fluid retention, weight gain may be two to five pounds, irritability and all the signs and symptoms of PMS result. (Remember the crazed cartoon cat with the caption "I have PMS and a handgun—any questions???")

Estrogen causes sensitive tissues to grow. It makes breasts larger and increases the thickness of the uterine lining. It stimulates the ovaries to produce cysts. As a result, if there is little or no progesterone around, these tissues are more likely to become cancerous. Birth control pills have been shown to increase a woman's chances later in life of developing cancer in sensitive tissues. Shortly after the introduction of Premarin, a huge increase in the incidence of uterine cancer prompted a search for a synthetic (there's that patent/profit issue again) analog of progesterone. The resultant inventions did reduce the incidence of uterine cancer, but they did not have any of the other effects of progesterone. They do not calm the brain, strengthen bones, assist in weight loss, or support healthy adrenal or thyroid function. They are a poor substitute for bioidentical progesterone. Progesterone—the real thing—is an anticancer hormone too. Mother Nature holds the patent.

Bones respond to this hormonal dance, too. Estrogen prevents bone breakdown, and it was the mainstay of osteoporosis treatment before the cancer scare and before the advent of the bisphosphonates, compounds like Fosamax that are derived from harsh chemicals akin to floor stripper. Progesterone actually promotes the formation of new, strong bone. I have seen increases in bone density of five to twenty percent as a result of progesterone supplementation over a period of several years. Progesterone can be taken for life.

Many women are self-treating with the progesterone cream that is being sold without a prescription in health food stores around the country. This is a step in the right direction. It misses the mark because these women cannot know if the progesterone in the preparation is adequate for their needs. Is it actually being absorbed? Is it stimulating the production of other hormones like estrogen, testosterone, or cortisol? Does my significant other need the dose he is getting when we cuddle? It is so important to get professional help in hormone replacement therapy, since these are powerful messenger molecules that you are likely to need for a very long time. Get tested once a year if you are using over-the-counter products, and see someone knowledgeable to monitor your response to treatment.

⤳⤳⤳⤝

The typical female patient arrives at the office in a state of agitation. She had carefully prepared her medical history, recent labs, and a list of questions to ask me, but she's left everything at home on the kitchen table. She got lost on the way to the office and arrives ten minutes late, apologetic. She refuses to be weighed. Her blood pressure and pulse are high. She sits down next to me and bursts into tears.

"Doctor Roberts, I don't know what's happening to me!" she wails. "I used to be so together—I could juggle home, the kids, my job, and a husband who really loves me but can't understand me at all! I don't even recognize myself anymore!"

She goes on to list her recent forgetfulness and irritability. She cries at commercials. She no longer has the patience to put together a meal and has gained fifteen pounds eating out every night. She once forgot her boss's name and she misplaces important papers. Her hair is falling out, she can't wear anything in her closet, and won't buy anything new because she's so ashamed that she's gone up two sizes.

While she's crying, I shake up a small bottle of progesterone in oil and ask her to open her mouth. I put three drops under her tongue, which, by the way, is red, cracked, and coated. I let her go on until she stops crying, and then I ask her to take a deep breath. I talk to her for ten minutes about how all this is a natural, if upsetting, manifestation of menopause. By the time fifteen minutes have passed, *she is smiling and laughing at her outburst. Progesterone has begun working its magic. We are on our way to a new, better life.*

THE RIGHT TIMING

Most women will do fine on progesterone alone until they reach late fifties or early sixties. During her forties and fifties a woman usually continues to produce enough estrogen, especially if she has a little bit of body fat. Often the first sign of needing estrogen is vaginal dryness. Intercourse becomes uncomfortable unless some kind of lubricant is used. Her mouth and eyes may be dry, her skin gets thin and flaky, and her memory goes. She wakes up in the middle of the night and can't get back to sleep. She needs estrogen, in addition to the progesterone. I usually give a low dose of estriol with a tiny bit of estradiol. Estriol is a "weak" estrogen that acts for twelve to fourteen hours. Estradiol will prevent hot flashes in the middle of the night, since it acts for twenty-four hours. Estriol is the safest of the human estrogens, and likely reduces breast cancer risk by 50%.[89] It's a great choice for older women. Sometimes a particularly estrogen-sensitive patient will do well on estriol alone given twice a day. Estriol is excellent for restoring vaginal lubrication and bladder health when given as a vaginal cream. Most women get near complete restoration of vaginal lubrication after one week of daily use, at which time the cream can be used every other day or every third day. The irritability and some of the incontinence of the menopausal bladder is greatly relieved as well. Overall, estriol is a safe and effective choice for women who might have a family history of gynecologic cancer. It is interesting that the FDA has chosen to ban bioidentical estriol in its transparent campaign to stamp out natural treatments of menopause. By its own admission, no adverse effect of estriol use *has ever been documented*. What's going on here? Women by the tens of thousands have been signing petitions,

8   "Estriol: safety and efficacy." Head, KA. Alt. Med Rev. 1998 April; 3(2):101-113.

9   "The bioidentical hormone debate: are bioidentical hormones (estradiol, estriol, and progesterone) safer or more efficacious than commonly used synthetic versions in hormone replacement therapy?" Holtorf K. *Postgrad Med.* 2009 Jan; 121(1):73-85. Review.

calling their Congress people and making their opinions known. The FDA has tapped the wrong segment of the population if they think that Boomer age women, educated and assertive as we have always been, will simply lie down and allow our hormones to be taken away? For no reason but the profit of some big drug company?? Come again??? Heads will roll, for sure, if this nonsense continues!

Once the major players progesterone and estrogen are in place and balanced, a saliva test or a urine collection is done, which may reveal the need for other hormones, namely DHEA, testosterone, and possibly cortisol. Many women will have good restoration of sex drive without these other hormones, but if the other hormones are low, they should also be given because they restore cellular and bone health, as well as benefiting libido. Hormone replacement is a lot like making soup—the spices may vary, but they must be balanced to get the right taste.

Repeat testing is done whenever the patient shows symptoms; for example, if she develops breast or nipple soreness or vaginal bleeding. Of course, any woman taking sex hormones should have an annual Pap smear if she has a uterus, once every three years if she has had a hysterectomy.

BREAST SCREENING – YOUR CHOICE

Breast exams should be performed and thermography or mammography done annually. A word about breast imaging: Mammography has been for decades the screening test of choice for breast cancer in the USA. In other countries such as New Zealand, Germany, France, etc., a different test is becoming more popular. This test is called digital infrared thermal imaging. It utilizes an infrared (heat) spectrum camera. Five views are taken of the chest, just like taking a photograph—no contact, no X-ray exposure. Heat inside the body, as from new blood vessels or high metabolic rate tissue, will light up as a hot spot. In this way very early cancers can be caught years before they would be visible on a mammogram. Since mammography has not been shown to extend life expectancy, and since X-ray exposure is cumulative and we are irradiating a sensitive body part year after year, many doctors prefer thermography for screening, with the mammogram reserved as a backup test if such is needed. But the need for manual evaluation of the breasts on a regular basis cannot be overemphasized. The person in the best position to do that is the patient. Good habits of self-examination are essential to keep the body in good condition and to alert a health provider should something suspicious arise.

HORMONES AND THE EMOTIONS

Hormone balance is very important for the health of a woman throughout her life. The close association of hormones with emotions is worth a mention here. For example, a high percentage of women experience sexual abuse at an early age, often at the hands of a family member or trusted friend. A lifelong mistrust of men and damaging self-hatred can be established and bring on problems that emerge throughout life. In an effort to protect herself from further invasion or indeed any type of sexual attention, a woman's subconscious mind may cause the body to accumulate excessive fat deposits. In my experience, most women with morbid obesity have a history of sexual trauma in childhood. Overcoming the weight issue must be accompanied by an exploration of the underlying abuse with the goal of shedding the lifelong emotional burden, along with the weight. Failure to undo the damage, embrace her sexuality, and rehabilitate the little girl will doom the most draconian weight loss strategies, including gastric bypass or stomach stapling. We are much more than our physical bodies, and failure to read the message in the morbidity means we lose the opportunity to heal fully at all levels. In fact, all illness comes from emotional imbalances and is the body's primitive effort to gain the conscious awareness that will heal the underlying emotional wound. Pay attention! You have the chance to change your life!

RECOMMENDED READING:

What Your Doctor May Not Tell You About Menopause. John R. Lee, MD, and Virginia Hopkins. Warner Books, 2004.

The Wisdom of Menopause: Creating Physical and Emotional Health and Healing During the Change. Christiane Northrup, MD. Bantam Dell, 2001.

Women's Bodies, Women's Wisdom: Creating Physical and Emotional Health and Healing. Christiane Northrup, MD. Bantam Books, 2006.

Menopause: A Spiritual Renaissance. Helene Leonetti, MD.

http://www.iact-org.org/index.html For information on thermography in general, and breast thermography specifically.

CHAPTER **9**

Effects of Environmental Toxins on the Body

"Man has lost the capacity to foresee and to forestall. He will end by destroying the earth."

—Albert Schweitzer

Aside from the issues associated with overspecialization and exclusive reliance on drug therapy, the biggest deficiency of conventional medicine today is the vast desert of ignorance surrounding the huge problem of environmental toxins.

In my med school days (thousands of years ago), there may have been some excuse for not including this topic in our curriculum. Today, with the vast accumulation of data relating to chemical toxicity, its ubiquity, its effects on the ecosystem, and the increasing knowledge of how these substances work on the body, there is no excuse, and yet this is a void still present in the training of physicians. It goes along with the de-emphasis on underlying causes of illness that characterizes modern medicine.

Part of the problem is political. Corporate, industrial America does not want to be held liable for people's illnesses. Since many disorders have multiple causes, including genetic susceptibility, it would be extremely difficult and costly to determine liability. Still, lawsuits such as the one instituted by Erin Brockovitch have been pressed, and have given hope to millions of people who feel they have been poisoned on the job or as a result of careless disposal of industrial waste. Millions more have been exposed to toxins in the course of military service. It is clear that the Bush administration chose to protect corporate interests over the health of individual Americans. We now have reason to hope for substantial change in the near future. Awareness has been rising and successes have been achieved, although too few and too slowly.

THE 800-POUND GORILLA – HEAVY METALS

This chapter will focus on some of the most damaging and the most common toxins in this country at this time. Much of the following information is considered controversial, but there is plenty of science that proves damage, and references are listed at the end of the chapter. The concerted efforts by corporations to keep this knowledge from the public, and the hobbling of governmental oversight agencies, have kept most of us in the dark about the effects of pollution on our lives. Even worse, this important knowledge is not even taught in most medical schools. It's the invisible 800-pound gorilla in the room!

Damage by heavy metal toxins is common and widespread. All of the world's oceans are polluted with mercury. If you eat fish, you are exposed to mercury (especially the big predator fish). If you have dental amalgam ("silver") fillings, you have continuous exposure every time you chew, brush, or have your teeth cleaned. When these fillings are removed, huge exposures can occur through vaporization, inhalation, and absorption of mercury across the membranes of the mouth and nose unless proper precautions are observed.

Mercury is known to be toxic before it is put in the mouth and after it is removed. How can it be OK when it sits in the teeth for decades? The American Dental Association has attempted to keep this fact under wraps, muzzling dentists and preventing them from discussing amalgam toxicity with their patients. So far they have behaved just like Big Tobacco did when the question of tobacco-caused illness was opened, in the 1980's. Many dentists have begun to quietly replace metal fillings with composite, a tooth-colored filling which is an acrylic compound used in cementing prosthetic joints in place. What the toxicities of that compound will turn out to be is anyone's guess, but hopefully it will be less than the known ill effects of mercury.

Mercury lodges in the liver, the kidneys, and the brain, where it binds with tissue proteins and sits there, generating "free radicals." These are highly charged particles which race about, pulling electrons and damaging all cell structures—proteins, cell membranes, DNA itself. It has been implicated in Alzheimer's disease, cancer, heart disease, dementia, childhood autism, ADHD, and many other conditions.

Lead is another heavy metal that's been in our environment for at least a century. It can be found in paint, solder, crystal, ceramic glazes, and many household items, including children's toys and some herbal medicines! The government keeps revising its advisory levels as to what is safe. Currently that level is 10 parts per billion (it started at 100ppb), but many scientists think that no level of lead is safe. Lead causes brain dysfunction, behavioral changes—aggression, depression, etc.—and lodges in the bone marrow where it interferes with the production of red blood cells, causing a characteristic pattern called "basophilic stippling" which can be identified on microscopic examination of the red blood cells. Anemia is a common indicator of lead toxicity. Lead deposits can sometimes be seen as "lead lines" on an X-ray of small bones, such as in the fingers.

Cadmium is a heavy metal found in cigarette smoke, auto exhaust fumes, power plant emissions, and many paint pigments. Secondhand smoke exposure can significantly raise cadmium levels in the body of a non-smoker.

> **The New York State legislature has banned the use of hair analysis as an adjunctive medical test.**

Hair samples from people who live in cities, for example New York, are often heavily laced with lead and cadmium. The characteristic aroma of the New York City subway is a heavy metal smell which millions are breathing every day. It is interesting to note that the New York State legislature has banned the use of hair analysis as an adjunctive medical test. What are they afraid of? (I've seen some hair tests of New York City residents and they are a fright—loaded with toxic metals! These tests have to be sent to the lab from outside the State of New York.)

Acute heavy metal poisoning can kill within hours. More common is the slow accumulation of numerous metals, over decades, from chronic low-grade exposure. Our bodies simply cannot excrete these metals, as they do not occur naturally and we have no mechanisms to deal with them. Most of the ailments of aging are due at least in part to heavy metal accumulation. These include fatigue, joint pain, anemia, cognitive decline, dementia, aggression, social withdrawal, loss of appetite, headaches, high blood pressure, digestive disorders, chronic sinus congestion, heart muscle weakness, and many other conditions.

CHEMICAL SOUP

P.C. dragged herself into the office two years ago, supported on both sides by her sister and brother-in-law, because she could barely walk. She weighed 84 pounds, 16 pounds under her normal weight, and appeared to be knocking on death's door.

A thorough history revealed that she owned a beauty salon, in which she had been working daily for fifteen years. Her health had begun to deteriorate for the past three years, and she was unable to find a doctor in Ohio, where she lived, to help her. Her sister was a patient of mine, and persuaded P. to come to Florida as a last resort.

We started her on vitamin-mineral IV's, since her digestion and assimilation was quite poor. Targeted nutrients to support detoxification were started, and she kept to a very clean, organic diet. Over the course of a summer she gradually regained strength and was able to return to Ohio, where she sold her business.

People who work in closed environments, breathing a lot of volatile (airborne) toxins all day, are exceptionally vulnerable to liver damage, especially if they lack one or more genes for detoxification, a fairly common problem. Tests are available for genetic markers and liver function. Identifying toxins is a difficult and expensive process, but in most cases it isn't necessary. If you support the body's detox processes and remove the constant inflow of problem compounds, the symptoms will usually resolve by themselves.

꙳꙳꙳

Each year tens of thousands of what nutritional physician Dr. Jonathan Wright would call "extraterrestrial molecules" are brought into use for all kinds of purposes. How many of them are tested before being introduced into our cars, our toys, our household furniture, our gardens? The answer is pitifully few, if any. How many of them wind up in our bodies? Hundreds, at the least. In one landmark study, the umbilical cord blood of ten newborn infants was tested for four hundred different chemicals. On average, each child has 254 of these chemicals already present, thanks to placental transfer from Mom. What subtle (and gross) physical, mental, and emotional changes will those chemicals cause that will affect their futures and those of generations to come?

No one can answer these questions at this time, but they will be answered eventually, should we survive as a species. Many of these chemicals are known to affect the reproductive system. We have seen frogs with two sets of sex organs, alligators with tiny useless penises, sperm counts of all sorts of animals (including people) on the decline for years.

This pattern of sexual mutation is also seen along the coastline in fish. Some scientists think it's a by-product of sunscreen runoff by bathers! What is that same sunscreen doing to our kids, who get lavish doses because we have become so chemical dependent that we have forgotten that a broad-brimmed hat and a shirt will protect from the sun too! Our sun phobia has led to a national epidemic of vitamin D deficiency, which predisposes us to osteoporosis, depression, cancer, and heart disease.

Another category of toxic chemicals is pesticides. Pesticides are carcinogenic in people. We pour them all over our gardens, our kitchens, and our golf courses. Nancy Nick, founder of the John W. Nick Foundation, advises golfers "don't lick your balls." Apparently this habit in her father, an avid golfer, may have led to his death from breast cancer. The Foundation is dedicated to raising the awareness of breast cancer in men, who comprise one in one hundred cases. (See www.JohnWNickFoundation.org)

Pesticides and fertilizer have created vast "dead zones" in the oceans. A huge one is in the Gulf of Mexico, where Mississippi River water carries tons of chemicals from the heartland of the country to dump into the Gulf. Fertilizer encourages algae bloom, which eats up the oxygen in the water, starving out other forms of life. This dead zone is estimated to be 88,000 square miles, about the size of the state of New Jersey, and is not the only one in the Gulf of Mexico.

INTERNAL COMBUSTION

In addition to ambient and occupational exposures, people under certain very common conditions are generating toxins in their own bodies.

One of the most common organisms in and on the human body is Candida. It is a family of microscopic yeast that lives on the skin and in the intestines. Yeast feeds on carbohydrates, especially the refined sugars and starches that are such a beloved part of so many people's diet. The yeast ferments these carbs, just as it would in the process of making beer and alcohol. Lo and behold! Alcohol and alcohol by-products (aldehydes) are the result. The person affected often describes their condition as a kind of "brain fog," along with fatigue and muscle and joint pains. Sound like a hangover? It should, it's the same chemistry, and it goes on day and night inside the gastrointestinal tract of the sufferer. It is especially common in people who have taken many courses of antibiotics or steroids (cortisone or similar drugs). Alternating constipation and diarrhea are common symptoms, as are bloating, tummy pain, and an addiction to sweets. These people may have skin rashes, especially in the creases of the body, sore tongues, which often have a coating of white fungus, and vaginal yeast infections that are uncontrollable (because the true reservoir is in the gut, and she's drinking Cokes all day). Not only does the yeast have to be treated, but the diet must change or the problem will happily recur whenever the sugar load is high enough.

FOOD ADDITIVES

One of the categories of invented chemicals that ought to be the best tested of any newly invented molecules is food additives. These should be proven safe before they go in any human being's mouth. This is the job of the Food and Drug Administration. Chemicals in this category include flavoring agents (e.g. MSG), colorants (FD&C#6), preservatives, emulsifiers, stimulants (like caffeine), artificial sweeteners, and others. MSG (mono-sodium glutamate) is remarkably similar to a naturally occurring amino acid, glutamate, which is highly active and concentrated in brain tissue. However, glutamate itself is neurotoxic in high doses, acting as an "excitotoxin." MSG is a flavor enhancer. It has no taste of its own, but it makes everything taste better, so it's put in almost every processed food. Anyone eating from boxes or cans, or anyone eating out, may be exposed to far more glutamate than exists in the natural food diet. The well-known "Chinese restaurant syndrome" includes tingling around the mouth, clenching of jaw muscles, and a strange sensation in the body. These are neurologic symptoms that occur from one large exposure at one meal. Chronic low dose exposure can cause excess stimulation of neurons which may lead to chronic neurodegenerative diseases like Parkinsonism and ALS (Lou Gehrig's Disease).

The following model of how illness develops is included here because it so aptly describes the onset and development of disease due to chronic toxin exposure and accumulation. It actually applies to the development of chronic disease from any cause.

RECKEWEG'S PHASES OF ILLNESS

In the late 1800s a physician by the name of Anton Reckeweg described the way an illness progresses. It can still help us understand the disease conditions that we see today. What is even more powerful, it can help us understand how to begin the process of "unwinding" or reversing the disease.

The first phase of illness happens in seconds to minutes of exposure to, say, a virus, a toxin, or an allergen. Phase one is **excretion**, or the production of large amounts of fluid in an effort to wash out the offending pathogen. This will result, depending on the organ involved, in diarrhea, excessive sweating, nausea and vomiting, a runny nose, or urinary frequency. It's the body's first defense. Minutes to hours later, phase 2, **inflammation**, sets in. This is when we develop rhinitis, bronchitis, gastritis, etc. Swelling and pain might accompany this phase. Tissues get red and swollen, and localized heat or systemic fever develops.

The next level of worsening brings us to the third phase, that of **deposition**. This is when the body attempts to wall off the offending pathogen by forming a polyp in the nose or the colon, or by growing a new wart on the skin. Uterine fibroids, fibrosis of the muscles, or lung tissue occurs. This phase generally takes days to months to develop.

So far all the action has taken place outside the cell membrane, on the surface of tissues, or in the spaces between the cells. The next three phases take place inside the cell. Phase four occurs over months to years and is called **impregnation**, and it describes the condition of chronic illness within the mechanism of the cell itself. It can cause asthma due to irritability of bronchial muscle tissue. It produces congestive heart failure or myopathy (failure of heart muscle to generate enough force to move blood efficiently through the body). Another condition called malabsorption happens when poorly functioning intestinal cells are unable to transport nutrients effectively, or are unable to effectively keep out substances that are harmful to the rest of the body. Here's also where the white blood cells begin to attack the tissues of the body in autoimmune disease.

Phase 5 takes years to decades to develop and is called **degeneration**. Conditions we think of as "normal aging" are included here, such as atrophic gastritis, in which the lining of the stomach no longer secretes acid or digestive enzymes and can't protect itself with the thick mucus lining that a normal healthy stomach would have. In the lungs this produces COPD – chronic obstructive pulmonary disease – or emphysema, which involves the loss of air sacs where oxygen is transferred from the breath to the body.

These conditions, while common, are by no means a necessary or normal part of aging.

Degeneration in bones is called osteoporosis, and arthritis when it involves loss of cartilage in the joints. In the liver it is cirrhosis, while in the brain it produces atrophy of the cerebral cortex, which often results in dementia.

The sixth and last phase of Reckeweg's progressive model of illness is **de-differentiation**, in which there are actual DNA mutations that occur over the course of decades. This results in irreversible changes in the cell, which either lead to actual cell death or to the development of cancerous changes.

The beauty of this model is that it shows where on a timeline of disease progression a person's illness might be. Even more exciting is Reckeweg's assertion that this process *is reversible* at any point in the continuum. The process can be interrupted and healing measures instituted at any point. In other words, there's always hope as long as you are this side of the grass.

Following the logic, when a person begins to heal, his disease process retraces the steps it took to get there. Providing supportive nutrients to a malabsorbing bowel will result in healing. However, the patient may have to endure swelling, inflammation, and diarrhea along the way, simply because the process requires retracing the path it took to get there. Normally, healing does not take as long as it takes to develop the illness. The natural tendency of the body is to push towards balance, and the body's mechanisms will restore themselves quickly if the impediment is relieved.

Another principle of healing according to homeopathic medicine (of which Dr. Reckeweg was a practitioner) is that disease progresses *from the outside in*. Skin and other surfaces are affected before the internal organs begin to show signs of damage. In the process of healing, the direction is reversed and recovery brings back old conditions. For example, a rash may disappear when hepatitis is active, but may reappear when the internal condition improves. Movement of symptoms from the inside to the outside is considered to be a good sign in homeopathic medicine.

So let's go on to what to do about pollution in your body.

RECOMMENDED READING:

Environmental Health. Dade Moeller, Professor Emeritus, College of Public Health, Harvard University, 1992, 1997, 2005.

Calculated Risks: The Toxicity and Human Health Risks of Chemicals in Our Environment. Joseph V. Rodricks, Cambridge University Press, 1992.

Silent Spring. Rachel Carson. Houghton Mifflin, 1962, 1990, 2002.

www.epa.gov Government website containing accessible information on pollution and food safety.

www.ewg.org Environmental Working Group website with up to the minute information on how to protect yourself and your family from environmental hazards.

http://www.healingfocus.org/Homotoxicology.pdf Article on the stages of illness and their treatment with homeopathy.

CHAPTER 10

Ridding the Body of Toxins

> **Clean up what's coming in,**
> **support the body's detoxification systems,**
> **eliminate the junk.**

Once you've realized how much your health is impacted by the existence of toxic substances in your environment, the next natural question is "What can I do about it?" The answer must begin with a little soapbox speech.

Until the world is cleaned up, any individual creature (human or otherwise) living in it cannot be pure. The oceans wash through each and every one of us, we are all breathing the same air, and the vandalizing of Mother Earth hurts all of her children. So think globally and act locally. We can and must clean up our act if we wish to be truly healthy.

Meanwhile, someone intent on doing the best he can will follow these steps: Clean up what's coming in, support the body's detoxification systems, eliminate the junk.

CLEAN UP THE INFLOW

Air, water, food, thoughts, and beliefs are rushing in and out of us all the time. Any asthmatic can tell you the quality of the air on any given day. He has a sensitive pollution meter in his chest. Many people can't leave the air-conditioned environment of their homes on some days in many cities around the world. But how does the average healthy person gauge the quality of the air, the water, and the food? Consider yourself fortunate if you have to ask the question.

Natural air is clean unless there's something pumping toxicants into it. Volcanoes and forest fires do that. Manmade pollution has added immensely to the level of particulates in the air. Agricultural areas for decades have used "crop dusting" as a technique for widespread application of pesticides. Coal-burning power plants are among the worst sources of pollution, spewing heavy metals and hydrocarbons into the air all the time. In many neighborhoods the cars are dusted with black soot every morning. **Don't stand under the crop duster** and **don't move in next to a power plant**. Likewise, in many areas of the country where there is a prolonged dry season and brush, or forest fires spring up all the time, the thick smog can be bad enough that people hundreds of miles away are coughing and choking on it. In some cities the winds don't blow the auto exhaust fumes away and the air has very low oxygen levels. Tokyo was the first city to offer "oxygen bars," where for a small fee you can breathe clean air through a hose. Now they exist in many places, including Miami, New York, and Cusco, Peru (high altitude is the reason here).

Protecting your lungs from polluted air is the first line of defense. If a sickening smog has taken over your part of the world, stay inside, or don't be too proud to wear a mask or bandana when you have to go out. Ultimately, you can move to a less polluted area.

ORGANS OF ELIMINATION

There are seven organs which carry waste materials out of the body. They are the colon, the kidneys, the skin, the lungs, sweat glands, lymphatics, and hair. The colon temporarily stores the body's solid waste on its way out. If waste material stays too long, water is reabsorbed back into the body, carrying with it water soluble toxins. Regular, soft, bulky movements keep this waste in contact with the bowel wall as short a time as possible, protecting the body.

The kidneys filter fluids and form urine, processing and purifying the blood. Each kidney is composed of masses of tiny capillaries arranged so as to excrete only certain chemicals, retaining those which the body still needs. For example, potassium is excreted while sodium is retained. Drinking plenty of clean water during the day is important for the kidneys to do their job. The electrolyte balance of the body is regulated by the adrenal glands. These two little glands produce aldosterone, a hormone that balances sodium and potassium levels in the blood.

The skin sheds its outer cells continually. In so doing, it can carry waste and toxins out of the body. This process of "exfoliation" can be assisted with vigorous scrubbing (with a loofah sponge or pumice stone) when the skin is warm and well hydrated, as during or after a bath. Stroking the skin from hands to heart, or feet to torso, assists the lymphatic system to push fluids back towards the heart where they can rejoin the blood and allow the excretion of toxins.

Lungs, of course, exchange gases in both directions. Many of our worst or most pervasive pollutants are carried into the body through the lungs and mucus membranes of the respiratory system. Particulate matter is filtered by the mucus-coated folds of the nasal passages. We have an opportunity to cleanse the nasal passages every day with use of a Neti pot. This device looks like a small Aladdin's lamp. It holds a small amount of salt water, which is used to wash the nasal passages. Simple mechanical cleansing can make a huge difference for the sinus sufferer. Deep breathing of unpolluted air brings fresh new oxygen into deeper pockets in the lungs and sweeps out stale old air.

♩♩♩♩

The Chinese say that the lungs are the seat of grief, and that old unresolved emotional wounds can show up as shortness of breath, chronic breathing problems, and tumors or cancers in this area.

♩♩♩♩

Sweat glands actively pump substances out of the body. They are responsible for large fluid and electrolyte losses in warm weather or with exercise. Hydration with electrolyte-containing fluids can be the key to restoring energy and keeping the body healthy. Sebaceous glands produce oils and waxy protectants that can move some fat soluble pollutants out of the body. Showering after exercise keeps the toxins from reabsorbing back through the skin.

Most people would include the lymphatic system as a waste processing plant, and this is correct. The lymph system collects fluids from outside the circulation and shepherds them back into the blood. In the process, impurities are filtered out by the lymph nodes. Because there is no pump (heart) in the lymphatic system, the upward movement of lymph fluid is accomplished through muscle contractions, i.e., exercise. Walking is an excellent activity to get these juices flowing. Massage directed at improving the flow of lymph can be very helpful in removing toxins from the tissues.

Hair is such a good recorder of toxicity that it was possible for modern-day scientists to analyze a lock of Beethoven's famously wild hair. They determined that the composer was actually killed by the steady administration of lead and mercury-containing medications by his physicians. Minerals are incorporated into the hair shaft, permanently recording what was in the circulation during the time that hair was growing. In about 50% of the population, heavy metals are effectively expelled by the body into the hair. The rest will have no toxins showing in the hair despite their presence in the environment and in the body. They are non-excreters. Therefore, the hair test is not always a good indicator of heavy metal toxicity. It can, however, in half the population, be an additional route of excretion of toxins.

FASTING

Fasting does not really mean starving yourself. It should simply mean a time-out from the normal digestive process. The best fasts provide essential nutrients and lots of water. Metabolic wastes and liberated toxins are still produced during a fast and need to be efficiently eliminated.

One of my favorite fasts can be done one day a week, or periodically for three to five days as a general "housecleaning" event. Here's the recipe:

Juice of three limes
Molasses or grade B maple syrup to taste
Cayenne pepper to taste
Water, about a quart

Blend all ingredients in a blender. Have as much as you want throughout the day. The limes provide vitamin C, the molasses some B vitamins and tasty sweetness, and the cayenne helps energize you and makes your stomach think there's something substantial in it. I like my evening portion ("dinner" if you will) to have some fiber, so I'll put 2 tablespoons of Metamucil or pectin in the blender with the other ingredients. That way everything keeps working smoothly and the toxins leave on schedule the next day.

HELP YOUR LIVER, PLEASE

There are certain foods and nutrients which are especially important for the detoxification process. These include high fiber foods (veggies), certain amino acids, minerals, and vitamins.

Fiber scrubs the walls of the intestines as it moves through. Fats and toxic chemicals will stick to the fiber and pass through without being absorbed. Fiber also traps water, making the consistency of stool softer and bulkier, therefore easier to pass. Certain intestinal bacteria (the good guys) feed on soluble fiber, so ingesting "pre-biotics" such as pectin will encourage growth of good bacteria.

THE LIVER – OUR CHEMICAL PROCESSING PLANT

The way the liver rids the body of metabolic waste, toxic chemicals, and used hormones is a two-step process. Phase 1 adds a reactive oxygen to the molecule, actually making it into a dangerous free radical. It is analogous to putting a hook on the wall so other things can be attached, but that hook can snag anything. This first phase of detoxification is a little tricky. If Phase 2 detoxification is impaired, these free radicals pile up and can damage the body more than the original chemical! It is therefore extremely important that the "conjugation" phase, Phase 2, be encouraged and supported. Some supportive nutrients are amino acids – **glycine,** sulphur containing… aminos like **cysteine**, **N-acetyl cysteine**, **glutamine**, and **methionine** are found in protein foods like eggs, chicken, fish, beef, and beans. They can also be taken as supplements if liver detox pathways are impaired or poor absorption is a problem. Sometimes sluggish reactions (perhaps due to acquired liver disease or genetic variations from normal function) can be pushed along by providing extra high amounts of materials for the body to work with.

Selenium is a mineral which is very important in detoxifying the body, since it binds mercury tightly and allows it to be excreted. It also powers up your vitamin E antioxidant. Selenium is found in onions and garlic.

Some foods make both Phase 1 and Phase 2 detox work better. Here comes the cabbage family again! **Indole-3-carbinol (I3C)** and **di-indole-methane (DIM)** are compounds that are beneficial for both components of this pathway. Because of that they are recommended for cancer treatment and prevention. The family includes cabbage, bok choi, kale, Brussels sprouts, broccoli, and cauliflower.

COLONICS

In India, yogis have always believed in internal cleansing as a general health maintenance procedure, just like tooth brushing or washing your hands. Colonics is the internal washing of the colon, similar to an enema but much more extensive.

A disposable insertion tube is gently placed in the rectum by a trained therapist (or by the person herself), which is attached to disposable tubing that conducts water into and out of the colon. The therapist opens a valve that allows water to flow gently in, massages the abdomen a bit, then allows the water to be expelled out again through the exit tube. Most systems include a glass-viewing tube so you and the therapist can actually see what's coming out. The process may take 30-60 minutes. It is not uncomfortable and is quite safe in the hands of a trained therapist.

Colonics will dislodge many things that the bowel itself has been unable to expel. Sometimes sticky substances will cling to the bowel wall and only come off with internal washing. People who are often constipated will find that the procedure stimulates better bowel function for weeks afterwards, since the bowel is cleaner and the muscles in the wall of the bowel function better as a result.

It seems a colon hydrotherapy machine would be a very useful piece of equipment to have in nursing homes and eldercare facilities, since older people often suffer from constipation. It could also be offered as an alternative way to cleanse the bowel before colonoscopy because it hydrates, rather than dehydrating the patient with diarrhea-inducing laxatives that are the current choice for bowel preparation.

SWEATING

Sweat is produced in order to cool the surface temperature of the body and allow the blood to dissipate a higher than normal internal body temperature. Sweat will also carry impurities out of the body. The smell of sweat varies greatly between individuals and even in the same individual at different times due to chemical and hormonal differences. It may even become a different color after exposure to dyes or pigments.

Exercise is one way to generate sweat. It is important for an athlete to remember to replace lost fluids and electrolytes like potassium and magnesium after a long race or practice session.

It is equally important to shower after exercise to wash toxins off the skin.

Another way to sweat it out is to use an infrared sauna. I recommend that cancer patients or people with sluggish detoxification pathways buy an individual sauna (They run from about $400 to $1,500) and use it for 30-60 minutes a day, or according to the manufacturer's directions.

BREATHING

The breath energizes and purifies the body. It has been used in yoga for centuries to access a state of relaxation. Physiologically and spiritually, the breath is fundamental to life.

Volatile compounds like ammonia and ketones leave the body through the breath. In the emergency room we can often diagnose a dangerous condition called diabetic ketoacidosis by the fruity odor of ketones on the breath.

Deep breathing, by blowing off extra carbon dioxide, will raise the pH of the blood, and can, after a few minutes, begin to cause a state similar to psychedelic hallucinations. The condition will self-correct in seconds after the deep breathing stops. Deep breathing controlled by a ventilator is used to decrease swelling inside the skull after brain injury. Slow voluntary deep breathing relaxes the nervous system and accesses a meditative state. Anxiety cannot coexist with slow deep breathing, so "toxic" thoughts can be banished with this technique.

CHELATION THERAPY

The procedure was invented to treat sailors who were poisoned by lead based paints used on battleships. The procedure involves the administration (by intravenous, oral, rectal, or transdermal routes) of a synthetic amino acid with several chemical binding sites. Chela- means "claw" in Greek, and refers to the ability of a compound to grab a metallic atom in a pincer-like grip. This quality allows the chelating agent to pull the metal out of storage in the bones, liver, kidneys, or the brain, and exit the body carrying the toxic metal with it.

Chelation therapy is the only FDA approved treatment for the removal of toxic heavy metals from the body, yet most doctors have little or no experience with it. If the subject of chelation arises, it is just dismissed with a wave of the hand and a terse "That's just quackery!" Most professors in medical school have never used it or researched it. The reason for this flippant attitude lies in the fact that chelation therapy has some "inconvenient" side effects. It happens to reduce calcium deposits in the walls of arteries. It can therefore reverse arteriosclerosis (hardening of the arteries). Many doctors' (and hospitals') livelihood depends on diseases of aging, and arteriosclerosis is one of the main causes of aging. A simple safe treatment like chelation therapy could make major heart surgery a thing of the past, reduce the incidence of stroke, and prevent and treat one of the underlying causes of cancer and dementia—metal toxicity.

TOXIC BELIEFS

> **This planet is a school, and we have come here to learn all we can about love, peace, and compassion.**

Not all toxins are chemical. Certain persistent thought patterns can be extremely deleterious to health, as well as to relationships. Constant mental chatter can be a never-ending loop of self-judging, angry, or depressive thoughts. This obsessive negative thinking wears grooves in the mind. Habits of mind can have extremely detrimental effects on the immune system. Many scientific studies have shown that negative emotions suppress immune function in many ways. People become sick more often, the numbers of white blood cells are affected, antibody production goes down, and so on.

The antidote is to *practice* (the operative word) positive thinking. Learn that happiness is a conscious choice. Let go of negative feelings. Resentments can be dissolved with forgiveness. Anger can eventually give way to compassion. Whatever was "done" to you can be viewed as a lesson that can bring a new level of understanding. It's called "the Cosmic 2 X 4." Instead of throwing blame bombs or pity parties, it might be more productive to ask yourself what you did—or did not do—to attract this painful learning. Did you not heed the warning signs? Every person you encounter in your life is a teacher for you, whether they know it or not. Even in the midst of an argument, you can listen for the nuggets of truth in what the other person is saying. A helpful attitude is to assume that *this planet is a school*, and we have come here to learn all we can about love, peace, and compassion. This is a healthy and life-enhancing attitude. You and those around you will benefit from the changes you are making. Perhaps they will be inspired to change, but that is not your concern. The only person you can change is you yourself. And this is your only job, your spiritual work. You came here to perfect yourself.

Meditation can be extremely helpful in gaining insight into and control over the process of thinking. The human mind is a power tool. It should not be encouraged to think it is in charge. The mind's true purpose is to work in service of spirit, and therefore it must be tamed. Your mind is a wild horse that has never been ridden. What is the most effective way to train a wild mind? Through firm, gentle, persistent effort—through meditation. Never get angry with yourself for losing your focus, be patient and persistent. Simply focus on one thing—your breath, a flame, a word. Keep pulling the mind back to that point of focus. After some time, maintaining focus will be easier and you will find yourself in better control of your thoughts—and your behavior—than you were before meditation. Meditation is one of the best things you can do for your health. It's free, it works, and you can do it anywhere (just like Kegel exercises)! Why not try? Toxic thoughts cannot live in a self-aware, calm, meditative mind.

HAVE THE COURAGE TO CHANGE YOUR LIFE

In the brilliant scheme proposed by David Hawkins, MD, PhD, a psychiatrist and mystic, levels of consciousness are ranked along a scale of 0-1000. Zero is dead—no consciousness. One thousand is God's perfect consciousness. Everything in between is possible to humans, if they choose a path of conscious self-improvement. You've already proven you are interested in conscious growth by reading this far in this book.

Levels from 1-199 represent the spectrum of negative thoughts. Fear is found here, as are shame, anger, frustration, low self-esteem, jealousy, laziness, and pride. Many people get sick because they spend too much time ruminating in a low emotional state.

In order to pull up into higher states of consciousness, a person must cross the demarcating line from negativity to possibility. The threshold state of level 200 is described by Hawkins as either **integrity** or **courage**. Integrity is the quality that makes it impossible to live a lie any longer, or to manipulate others. Without courage there is no growth beyond the known.

Passing that 200 milestone is the gateway to greater and higher levels of consciousness. From here, the level of 300 represents **detachment**, a benign quality that allows for action or inaction without the pressure of emotion. It doesn't mean coldness, it simply means detached awareness. Think of the Dalai Lama, who has more reason than most to be angry or sad. Instead, he is a living example of detachment (300) and compassion (which calibrates at 600 and higher).

The level of 400-499 is where the **rational mind** rules. Clear thinking, logic, analytical processes, and the scientific method occur here. This is why the rational mind can never understand **love**, which calibrates at 500-599. Love looks like madness to the mind. Love is actually the "logic" of the heart. Love is not limited to romantic attachment, but also friendship, love of humanity, love of God, and love of self as a manifestation of God. **Compassion** ranks 600 on the scale of consciousness. Unconditional love with empathy and the selfless desire to serve are found here.

Over 700 are the states of consciousness of the enlightened beings, the prophets, the avatars. Those are people who live to serve, to bring a message to humanity, to maintain the vision of a better world to come.

The Hawkins scale of consciousness is a roadmap for personal growth. Learning requires the faculty of **conscious awareness**, a quality that changes a person from a sheep to a self-directed student of life. This path is not easily taken, as self-responsibility can be scary and fear is a paper tiger many people are not willing to face. For the ones who do walk through the crucible, the reward is great. Life is more free, more open to possibility, and one finds that fear is an invisible barrier. It does not exist once you've walked through it.

In fact, life is about growth, from start to finish. Growth and learning are not just for schoolchildren; they are a natural and essential function of life and are arguably the most rewarding of any human activity.

RECOMMENDED READING:

Power vs. Force. The Hidden Determinants of Human Behavior. David Hawkins, MD, PhD, Hay House, 1995, 1998, 2002.

Toxic Metal Syndrome: How Metal Poisonings Can Affect Your Brain. H. Richard Casdorph and Morton Walker, 1995.

Detoxification and Healing: The Key to Optimal Health. Sidney MacDonald Baker, MD, 1997.

Detoxification - All you need to know to recharge, renew and rejuvenate your body, mind and spirit! Linda R. Page, ND, PhD, Traditional Wisdom, 1999-2002.

Encyclopedia of Homeopathy. Andrew Lockie, Dorling Kindersley Publishers, Ltd., 2006.

Everybody's Guide to Homeopathic Medicines. Stephen Cummings, MD, and Dana Ullman, MPH, Jeremy P. Tarcher/Penguin, 1997, 2004.

CHAPTER **11**

Sex - Keeping It Up Longer

"Many men die at 25 and aren't buried until they are 75."

—Benjamin Franklin

♪♪♪

**"Before sleeping together these days,
people should boil themselves."**

—Richard Lewis

One of the scariest aspects of getting older is the prospect of losing one's sex drive, being unable to perform, or not being attractive to a partner.

There are three things required to remain sexy well into "old age"—hormone balance, a functional brain, and a functional body. (See the rest of this book.)

♪♪♪

Motivation for sex changes as one ages. For men, the rutting instinct is extremely strong in his twenties and thirties and often beyond. Settling down with a single partner may bring a certain staleness and boredom, while pursuing multiple partners throughout life may lose its newness as well, not to mention exposing oneself to the risks of sexually transmitted diseases or harm at the hands of a jealous husband!

For some people, the sheer fun of exploration with different partners can be a motivator. Others seek the temporary boost to self-esteem that sex can confer. Most people find that sex is an emotional bonding experience. Sex is, of course, the way we make babies, cement families, and grow partnerships that are intended to last a lifetime. As we have seen, hormones accompany feelings, and love is no exception. Oxytocin is the orgasm hormone in women. It is also the hormone involved in falling in love. Interestingly, it is also the hormone that initiates labor when the baby is ready to be born. One might say it's the Big Bang molecule itself!

Relationships are crucial to personal growth, no matter what form they take. By the time we reach our fifties, sixties, or older, we have explored (or opted out of exploring), we have tasted (or not), and most of us have settled into a much slower rhythm of desire. Still, it is not necessary to give up sex, or settle for less satisfying sex, or cease to enjoy the sheer fun of it. But the focus has changed.

One more face lift and
she'll have a beard!

A good laugh and a good cuddle is sometimes all you can do, but these activities can cement a relationship more than the acrobatics and extreme sports of youthful sex. It's the feeling that counts. Getting close to one another is delicious. Letting down one's guard is a great relief, so judgment can't be part of the process, especially self-judgment. One of the best assets one can have in elder sex is a good sense of humor. As bodies inevitably droop, or bloat, or crinkle, it helps to be able to laugh at ourselves to get over the embarrassment of all that.

The biggest "payoff" of sex (beyond its biological purpose) is the potential for transcendence that exists in the realm of sexual relations. It is possible to ride the energy of sex all the way to enlightenment. Tantra is the yogic science of sensuality as a spiritual practice. It involves seeing your partner as a specific manifestation of Creation itself, to make love as if the Goddess Herself is your partner. What woman wouldn't respond to that? But that's an attitude that takes a certain spiritual maturity. Why not try something new tonight?

❧❧❧❧

I once had a dream, when I was still quite young and juicy, that I was making love with an old man I'd never met in waking life. His skin was a deep mahogany black, he had a grizzled white beard, and he was very thin and very old, like Picasso's guitar player. Still, he made love to me in the sweetest, most erotic way, slowly and reverentially, as if holding the Queen of the Nile in his hands. I never forgot the feeling of being touched in that way. It happens so rarely in real life.

❧❧❧❧

Another dream involved a man I lusted for, although both of us were married to other people and were not willing to act on our feelings. Doubtless for that reason, the intensity of the desire was overwhelming. The dream had me walking up a hill where he was literally hanging on a cross. I spread my arms too, and as I approached him, sparks of lightning shot from me to him and back again. We never touched, in the dream or in real life.

❧❧❧❧

The controversial guru, Bhagwan Shree Rajneesh, was controversial partly because he thought sex is a good thing, even for people on a spiritual path. He saw sex as the Tantric ladder one could climb to experience the divinity in ourselves. This is a synopsis of what he said. A sexual relationship involves the merging of chakra energy. The concept of "soul mates" is real. It happens when two people are connected through all seven chakras. Although very rare, it can happen. It is as if the two are truly one person. They think alike, feel alike, and when they make love it is a cosmic merging on a parallel with the greatest transcendent experience you can imagine. It is coming home. It is like being back in the womb with your identical twin.

If only six centers are connected, also extremely rare, the feeling is no less. There is a delicious tension present in the one center that does not connect. It is self and other that is merging, not two identical souls, but two souls different enough from one another that there is space between them. Still, the harmony and joy is overwhelming, combined with the subtle thrill of one chakra out of synch. When two centers are different, or three, the polarities are more pronounced. The sex may still be great, but the potential for misunderstandings and friction is greater. For liaisons involving one or two chakras, this does not bode well for long-term stability. There may still be excitement in the coupling, but more likely than not, there will be too many differences for a relationship to last. These pairings often involve a one-night stand or a very short-term romance.

As we age and gather experience with all sorts of relationships, we can be more discriminating in our choices. No longer is the biological need so strong. This is a good time to learn the techniques of Tantric sex. Tantra uses sexual energy in a spiritual context. By picturing the partner—and oneself—as a manifestation of the Divine—a god or a goddess—sex becomes a cosmic event. Through breathing and meditation, facing one another, the sexual energy is allowed to build in a slow and steady way, before any touching begins. This energy is moved upwards through breathing and visualization, perhaps without touching the partner at all, until it ultimately climaxes all the way up to the seventh chakra. Orgasm is total involvement of body and soul, with simultaneous transcendence of the physical. A man normally loses energy when he climaxes. In Tantric sex the man does not ejaculate, or if he does, the semen is discharged internally, pushing the freed energy right back into the body. A woman gains energy with orgasm, and so is encouraged to have multiples. All this is done by mentally equating the beloved with the Goddess or the Divine. How different from the sweaty rutting that many of us have grown accustomed to!

Humans are a strange lot. We are the only members of the Earth family who have made a fetish of sex. Sex has so many complicating emotional and psychological meanings that it has become unrecognizable as a biologic function. Other animals are much more matter-of-fact about it. In the bonobo chimp society, for example, sex is how they say hello—they have sex with everyone, male-female, male-male, and female-female. Perhaps because of this constant expenditure of energy, the bonobo is the most peaceful of the great apes. They rarely exhibit aggression, and solve their conflicts with a roll in the hay instead of fisticuffs. Their food source is plentiful, and because anyone can couple with anyone else, there is no fighting over mates. So could our human proclivity for violence simply be frustrated sexuality in disguise? If we were a more open society in terms of sex, would we be less warlike? Is it possible that we might be able to give up war as a means of conflict resolution and resolve our disputes with a friendly diddle instead? Were the flower children of the 1960s on to something when they suggested that we "Make love, not war"? On the other hand, if we were more open sexually, would we still be here? We might be even more vulnerable to sexually transmitted plagues, diseases, and jealous rages.

Our challenge now is to find a way out of our pain and our reflexive violence. When will hurting each other be understood to be as foolish as a liver attacking a heart, or a skin cell declaring war on the blood? What can we do instead of killing each other to prove a point? Historically, games and competition have always functioned as a substitute for violence. The players are our gladiators on one level, but on the other hand, team identification is another thing that divides us, in a more or less friendly way. In designing the New World, we will find new games to play. They are more likely to be games that require cooperation, like team treasure hunts or neighborhood clean-ups made fun.

**"The path to enlightenment is long –
Bring a sandwich and a magazine."**

—Issy Lambeck

Action points for staying sexually active into old age:

- hormone balance (Chapter 8)
- exercise to keep your heart strong and your mind flexible
- nutrition that doesn't clog your arteries
- Chelation therapy (see Chapter 10)
- Constant detoxification of physical and emotional poisons

CHAPTER 12

Other Forms of Treatment

In facing the difficult choices one has to make when illness strikes, or in simply deciding how to stay well, it is helpful to know what is available to you and to understand something about the different "modalities" of treatment.Following are some of the most important and the most accessible treatments you might want to use. For all but the last of these, there is peer-reviewed science supporting the safety and usefulness of the treatment. This list is not complete and leaves out many excellent treatments, but the ones included are all modalities I have some experience with and therefore feel comfortable recommending.

ACUPUNCTURE

In Traditional Chinese Medicine (TCM), one of the best-known forms of treatment is acupuncture. This involves the placement of fine needles in certain well-defined points along the energy meridians of the body. (See Chapter 3 for a discussion of energy anatomy.)

As in all modalities in TCM, the goal is to balance the energy flow (chi) in the body. A well-placed needle will relieve an energy block, energize a weak flow, or decompress trapped chi. Since each of the fourteen meridians is connected to internal organs, this superficial needling can have profound effects on internal functions.

Conditions that have been shown to be helped by acupuncture are pain, chronic fatigue, inflammation, anxiety, headache, muscle tension, stress, depression, and many others. This astonishing treatment first came to the American public's attention when James Reston, editor of *The New York Times*, accompanied President Richard Nixon on his historic first trip to China. As luck would have it, Reston developed appendicitis and was treated in a Chinese hospital. The operation was done—same as in the States—in the usual way under general anesthesia. However, postoperatively he received, not pain pills, but acupuncture. Its effectiveness in controlling his pain was remarkable, and the stage was set for acupuncture to make its appearance in the USA. Now, thirty-five years later, every town has its acupuncture clinic, and this modality is no longer thought to be strange.

CHIROPRACTIC

In 1987 the AMA lost a restraint of trade lawsuit against the chiropractic profession. As a result, the AMA was forced to print a statement in its publication *JAMA* that chiropractic is "more effective than conventional treatment" for acute back pain. This verdict was supposed to have ended the harassment and marginalization of the profession of chiropractic by the medical establishment. Still, chiropractic is rarely, if ever, given any credence by conventional medicine, and is generally disparaged by most medical doctors. Nevertheless, insurance usually covers chiropractic treatment.

Chiropractors are trained to relieve internal conditions through manipulation of the spinal column. The theory is that the spinal nerves, which control much of what goes on in the body, are pinched, stretched, or otherwise distorted by slight irregularities in the way the vertebra stack up, one on top of the other. By correcting these misalignments, the nerves are released and ill health and discomfort are relieved.

Many, but not all, chiropractors, are knowledgeable about nutrition, detoxification, and other adjunctive therapies.

FLOWER ESSENCES

In the late 1800s in England, a physician named Edward Bach (pronounced "Bock") observed and enjoyed the natural world around him. He followed the life cycles of various plants, and theorized about how they mimicked human traits. Because he believed that all things in nature have a purpose for humanity, he developed what have come to be known as the Bach Flower Essences. He would pick the flower, the most potent expression of that plant's life, float it in a bowl of pure water, and set it in the sunshine. The information contained in that flower would permeate the water, so that when the flower was removed, the flower's "essence" remained. Clearly, these are energy remedies, which carry information in vibrational form, as opposed to chemical treatments like our pharmaceutical drugs, nutritional supplements, or herbs.

Flower essences are sold in health food stores and on the Internet. Nowadays, many more essences are available besides the 38 Dr. Bach discovered. They come from all over the world and can be used for many conditions. Most often they are used to treat emotional or psychological imbalances. For example, the essence **Star of Bethlehem** is given to someone who is paralyzed by grief, to give him hope. **Elm** is a useful essence for a person who is mentally and physically exhausted. And the combination **Rescue Remedy** can be used to calm a person about to take a test, restore function to someone traumatized by an accident, or even, as I sometimes do, to bring peace to two frisky puppies fighting with each other. Many women carry Rescue in their purses, since it is so handy for sudden unexpected challenges!

The flower essence is usually preserved with alcohol. Several drops can be placed directly on the tongue, or in a glass of water, then sipped slowly. Diluting the essence does not diminish its potency. It can be rubbed on a paw or on a baby's nose, and it will still work.

Flower essences are one of the best "guerilla" modalities available to people for home use. They are meant for emotional blockages and are safe for children and pets. They have no interactions; that is, they can safely be given with other medications, and they have no side effects. Think of their effect in the same way that a song can change a bad temper. The energy pattern of a particular flower essence will act on your emotions the way the right song can bring you out of a bad mood.

HERBAL MEDICINE

This venerable treatment modality is the way all indigenous peoples have treated sickness since long before recorded history. Local plants have always been used as medicine to heal wounds, treat fevers, and make people fall in love. During the Dark Ages in Europe, millions of herbalists and healers were put to death as witches because they represented the "pagan" paradigm. The emerging Church could not share the stage with the powers of Nature, and so these healers, midwives, and shamans had to go. So did the knowledge of herbal medicine that they had amassed over thousands of years. Today, we are exploring once again these gifts of Nature. The drug industry itself looks to the forests and jungles for new drugs, and people all over the world are growing medicinal herbs in window boxes and backyards. In many countries, food and spices are recognized for their ability to heal—from Grandma's chicken soup to the elaborate structure of Ayurvedic medicine in India, which rightfully makes food the cornerstone of good health. Many time-honored remedies have been dismissed as "old wives tales," but these old wives were the backbone of healing throughout many hundreds, if not thousands, of years, and we are now attempting to rediscover what they knew. The following few examples are intended to be illustrative, since a more complete discussion is beyond the scope of this book.

- **Stinging Nettles** – This sharp, spiny weed grows all over North America. It is used to reduce inflammation and to stop allergic reactions. Nettles tea, or tincture, or capsules of the powdered dried leaf can be purchased at any health food store and are an excellent substitute for antihistamine medication. Nettles does not dry the membranes of the mouth and nose and does not cause drowsiness.

- **Chamomile, valerian, lavender, hops, passionflower** – all well researched to be calming to the mind and a great help in inducing sleep.
- **Papaya, pineapple –** enzymes in these foods assist in the digestive process. The whole foods aid digestion, but most often the specific enzymes **papain** and **bromelain** are isolated from these fruits and used in combination with other substances.
- **Comfrey, hyssop** – can be used topically for healing wounds. Extracts may be applied directly (not tinctures, which contain alcohol and would be painful) or a tea made and used as a compress.

One of the most remarkable uses of herbal medicine is a practice in use all over the jungle areas of South America. This combination brew is called "yage," or "ayahuasca"—meaning "the vine of the dead." It consists of the bark of the vine, plus leaves from a second plant containing DMT, a powerful hallucinogen. A component of the bark prevents the breakdown in the stomach of this vision-inducing compound. The brew is carefully concocted by specially trained shamans. It is taken in the context of a sacred ceremony. The "spirit of ayahuasca" is personified. It is said to answer any question put to it, including how to heal sick people and how to navigate the higher spiritual dimensions. Most ayahuasqueros (the shamans who use the brew) say that it has taught them all they know about the properties of the plants around them. They call it "Doctor Ayahuasca" and insist that it can only do good. "Doctor Ayahuasca is 100% medicine," said our shaman, who had worked with the plants for 38 years in the Peruvian jungle.

HOMEOPATHY

One of the safest and most effective forms of alternative treatment is a type of medicine called homeopathy. In the Victorian era, homeopathy was widely used in the United States. However, the last school of homeopathic treatment was closed in the 1950s, due to pressure from the AMA and no doubt the emerging drug companies which couldn't tolerate the efficacy of these safe, inexpensive treatments.

Homeopathic remedies are taken from the natural world. They may be animal, vegetable, or mineral in origin. A remedy is prepared as follows: One part remedy is dissolved in 99 parts (or 9 parts, depending on whether you are making a "c" or an "x" dilution) of solvent (water or alcohol). The solution is shaken hard for a given length of time ("succussed") before one cc is withdrawn and diluted into another 99cc's of water. The new dilution is succussed again. This process is repeated over and over. After about 7 dilutions, the solution contains not a molecule of the original substance. The "potency" of a remedy is indicated by a number placed after the Latin name of the original substance. For example, the remedy **coffea cruda 30c** is made from raw coffee, diluted 30 times over in a 1:100 ratio. This is considered a relatively low-potency remedy, as dilutions can go up to 1000 or higher. Lower potency (6, 12, 30) remedies work mostly on the physical body. Higher potencies help with mental, emotional, and even spiritual healing. Homeopathy is energy medicine. It works, not on the chemical processes of the body, but rather as a vibration that helps bring the patient's energy field back into correct relationship with itself and the larger environment. It would be similar to playing a happy song to someone who is suffering. The song can be played over and over (repeat dosing) until the person comes out of their depression and starts dancing. At that point the remedy (and the song) is no longer required, but may be repeated as needed for relapses. The right remedy for a particular condition is very specific. It will treat a symptom picture that at full strength, would cause the symptoms you are treating. In other words, "like cures like." In our example, drinking strong coffee causes mental alertness and busy mental chatter. Many people suffer from inability to fall asleep because their minds are too active and they don't know how to shut off the chatter. **Coffea cruda** is the perfect remedy for this exact condition.

In the same way, **Ipecac**, used in emergency rooms to induce purging, is a homeopathic remedy for nausea and vomiting. **Arsenicum album** is a remedy for food poisoning, vomiting, and diarrhea, and for burning pain anywhere in the body, symptoms that would be caused by arsenic itself. There are thousands of remedies. There is only one "constitutional remedy" that fits a person's energy signature and will bring that person back to "normal" no matter what the problem. However, many different remedies can be used in specific situations for specific issues.

The remedies can be purchased in health food stores. They consist of small pellets, usually lactose based (not enough to cause a problem even in lactose intolerant people). Two or three of the tiny pellets are placed under the tongue and allowed to dissolve there. If the situation is acute, re-dosing can be done every five minutes, until relief is attained. If after six doses nothing has happened, try another remedy. Some companies make combination remedies designed to alleviate certain symptoms and containing several individual remedies. This makes it easy for the novice to select something that will work, without knowing the remedy picture of each of the thousands of possible treatments. The combination remedies are usually named for the condition they are supposed to treat, such as "Sinus" or "Chest Cold," etc.

Homeopathy usually has no side effects, no interactions with drugs or supplements, and is a great home remedy for even the youngest children and for pets. Of course, if a child is too sick and doesn't respond quickly to the remedy, take him to a doctor or an emergency room. Western medicine has its definite strengths. Giving a remedy en route to the ER may help enough that the child avoids a hospital stay.

ENERGY MEDICINE

In recent times this most ancient of healing systems has been resurrected. The term covers a multitude of modalities, but all work with the human energy field. Actually, all forms of natural medicine work with the human energy field, but "energy medicine" does so directly and intentionally.

Some energy practitioners work with sensitive electronic equipment that measures vibrational frequencies and calculates what will bring the system into harmony again. Other practitioners use their hands to transmit a powerful wave that can often be sensed by the patient (as heat or a tingling sensation), which works in the same way. Some use their psychic abilities to read a person's energy and identify energetic problems that need fixing. They speak of "holes" in the aura, "weak" chakras, "low chi," or "entities" in the energy field that drain the person's vital flow. They can help the person travel back in memory to the origination point of the problem, and fix it!

A friend of mine, Oly, a medical intuitive, works in this way. She was asked to consult (by telephone) in the case of a three-month-old infant who was literally near death. The child would not eat. By "consulting" with the child's spirit guides, Oly discovered that the child did not want to be in a body, fearing its parents never wanted him to be born. In fact, when the pregnancy was first discovered, they had debated getting an abortion. When the parents were made aware, they began reassuring the child through holding it and cradling it and singing to it that it was truly welcome in this world. The child responded almost immediately and the "depression" quickly lifted. (How many children feel they are not really wanted?)

Many of these modalities do not require the patient and practitioner to be in the same room, or even the same country! Through the concepts of quantum physics, we now have a framework for understanding and testing seemingly magical treatments. Distant healing, intercessory prayer, healing touch, and others have been investigated by science and found to have some validity. Science is catching up with the old wives, and soon we will all understand that we are energy beings in a physical body.

Transferring healing energy from one person to another has been validated as a therapeutic tool. Sometimes special symbols are used, as in Reiki. Sometimes a physical substance can absorb the love and care that went into the making of it, as with Grandma's chicken soup or a specially charged crystal. Energy transfer can also be direct, person-to-person, as in Therapeutic Touch, Quantum Touch, or "the laying on of hands."

ASTROLOGY

> *In the same way that the full moon draws the waters of the earth toward itself, so do all the planets and constellations bring out tendencies that lie latent within us.*

Since we are already out on a limb, let me put in a word for an ancient art that still has much to offer us.

Ancient cultures all over the world spent countless hours studying the night sky. They personified and tried to make sense of the arrangements and the movements of the lights in the sky. Today we call this science "astronomy." The sister to astronomy is the art of astrology, which works with the energetic resonances from the heavenly bodies that impact our lives. Imagine yourself in a great cathedral, listening to the sounds of a huge organ as it plays a grand hymn. You feel the vibrations in your bones, your mind is elated with the beauty of it, and your spirit soars. Now imagine that instead of an organ, we are able to hear the vibrational frequencies of the planets and stars themselves. The way they interact and resonate at the moment of your birth becomes "your song," or your birth chart. These particular harmonies and dissonances will be a part of you for life, representing the strengths and weaknesses unique to you. Current positioning of the cosmic carillon in the sky activates different parts of your birth chart. Astrology therefore is very helpful in determining the timing of important events, and in assessing if two individuals will harmonize or clash energetically.

In the same way that the full moon draws the waters of the earth toward itself, so do all the planets and constellations bring out tendencies that lie latent within us. Astrology is not a just a predictive tool (although it can be used that way); it is a map that one can use as a guide to events and timing in one's life. Its usefulness, as in all modalities, depends on the skill and knowledge of the practitioner. I have had the great honor of befriending a professional astrologer of more than 60 years. Betty has taught me, through her great proficiency and counseling abilities, to respect this ancient art, which has guided empires past and present.

FURTHER READING:

www.NCCAM.nih.gov - The official website of the National Center for Complementary and Alternative Medicine, very easy to access and find information about most treatment methods.

The Web That Has No Weaver. Ted J. Kaptchuk. Contemporary Books, McGraw Hill, 2000. 2nd edition. Chinese medicine explained.

Between Heaven and Earth: A Guide to Chinese Medicine. Harriet Bienfield and Efrem Korngold. Another readable introduction to Chinese medicine.

Principles and Practices of Chiropractic. Scott Haldeman and Scott Haldeman. McGraw Hill, 2005.

The Complete German Commission E Monographs. Edited by Mark Blumenthal. German government official position papers based on scientific research on herbs as medicine.

PDR for Herbal Medicines, 4th edition. Thompson Healthcare, New Jersey, 2007. Reference book on herbs, their uses, side effects, and interactions with medicines and other herbs from the *Physician's Desk Reference* people.

The Way of Herbs. Michael Tierra, Pocket Books, Simon & Schuster, New York, 1998.

Consciousness, Bioenergy and Healing: Self-Healing and Energy Medicine for the 21st Century (Healing Research, Vol. 2; Professional Edition) by Daniel J. Benor, MD. Wholistic Healing Publications, Medford, NJ, 2004.

Everybody's Guide to Homeopathic Remedies. Stephen Cummings, MD, and Dana Ullman, MPH, Jeremy Tarcher/Penguin, New York, 2004.

Practical Homeopathy. Vinton McCabe. St. Martin's Griffin, New York.

A Practical Guide to Vibrational Medicine: Energy Healing and Spiritual Transformation. Richard Gerber, MD, HarperCollins, 2000.

Radical Healing: Integrating the World's Great Therapeutic Traditions to Create a New Transformative Tradition. Rudolph Ballentine, MD, Three Rivers Press, New York, 1999.

Hands of Light. Barbara Brenner, RN, Bantam Books, 1987.

The Astrologer's Handbook. Frances Sakoian and Louis Acker. Harper Resource Book.

Astrology for Spiritual Fulfillment. Jan Spiller and Karen McCoy. Simon & Schuster, New York, 1988.

CHAPTER 13

The Big, Bigger, Biggest Picture

"Today for you, tomorrow for me."

—Inca shamanic saying

The truth is that no matter how hard you work at getting and staying healthy, the context in which you perform this struggle will support or will sabotage your best efforts. Concentric circles of influence surround the individual—family, work, society, religion, planet—and impact directly on the well-being of every one of us.

Within the family unit, where there is not respect and equality, there is imbalance. Equality does not mean everyone is the same, or contributes in the same way, but rather that the contribution of each is valued equally and the input of each is equally important. The job of the "stay-at-home mom" is arguably the toughest and most important job on the planet. But it is usually funded by the "go-to-work" father. Supportive spouses help each other find time to exercise, meditate, and cook healthy meals. Passive-aggressive behavior on the part of a resentful partner must be confronted in order to make space for personal growth.

Our capitalist, materialist system, while allowing for unequalled individual freedom, is excessively tipped towards "every man for himself." Extended families are no longer the rule, but rather the exception. The old neighborhoods where kids played in the street all day, neighbors keeping an eye on everyone's kids, not just their own, functioned like extended families at one time. But the extreme mobility of our population and the tendency to move frequently make us strangers to the folks next door. Elderly people die in their homes and are not found for days because they never have visitors and no one cares enough to check on them. Loneliness and the fear of dying alone shadow all of us. Oak trees in Florida remain standing through a hurricane because their roots are intertwined under the earth. We miss a connection to a community, whether family or neighborhood, and our individual growth may be stunted by lack of it. Shared support systems work cooperatively. As the Inca shamans say, "Today for you, tomorrow for me."

On a larger scale, war grows from the smallest scars in our own hearts—anger, fear, resentment—to become the collective horror of violence of one people on another. Unspeakable abuse perpetrated by humanity on the animal kingdom, wild and domestic, is another aspect of our inability to see that we are all one. The interconnectedness of life is a concept that can heal our historic hatreds. We must illuminate the web that connects us all.

The violence we perpetrate on each other is no worse than the violence we do to our home planet. Gaia is a lovely, generous, supportive, and (most of the time) gentle Mother Earth who holds us to her breast, feeds, waters, and clothes us. On top of this, she gives us the completely gratuitous bonus of the incredible beauty of the Earth in her natural state.

The sight of the waters of the earth polluted and stinking, the great trees chopped down for toilet paper, the land itself stripped and mined for minerals, or in the course of war, laced with land mines—this is a sin. The way we treat our Mother will determine our fate.

As we approach the day of reckoning, which the Mayans predict in 2011-12, we must know that the wounds of the earth and all of her children are carried in the blood and bones of each one of us. As long as the least among us is suffering, we all suffer. We are interconnected in such a way that we depend upon each another. At this pregnant time in history, we have an opportunity to make the next evolutionary leap. We can realize the truth that we are in reality one organism, children of God, indivisible. You don't see one hand fighting the other, or a kidney refusing to work with a bone or a bladder or a brain. We humans have constructed a "nervous system" for our planet called the Internet. We have a complex circulation (transport) system that brings nutrients and commodities to and from every point on the globe. We interact socially, economically, politically—yet we have so far been unable to overcome our ancient addiction to violence against each other. Now is the time to grow up and stop all that childish nonsense!

The remedies for all our planetary ills may not be known yet, but the path ahead must include at least the following fundamental shifts in thinking and behavior:

1. **This planet is alive**. We depend on her for our life. We must relearn the proper respect and behaviors toward our Mother Earth. We are part of this system too.

2. **Women must be respected** as well, for the uniqueness they possess, their contributions to home, family, economy, politics, the arts, etc. The biological function of women as baby factories is a great thing. But all women and men too can contribute in other, no less meaningful, ways to the good of all if the good of all were more important to us.

3. Marginal societies, marginalized people, and the **poor of all nations** will be allowed a place at the table. They **must be afforded opportunities** to create better lives, to sustain themselves, and to become productive, respected members of a global society.

4. The **plants and animals** of the Garden are our wards. They too **must be respected and protected**, if we are to survive.

5. **Clean, renewable, non-polluting sources of energy** must be allowed to replace the current dependence on dirty

fossil fuels. Status quo power and wealth must not be allowed to stifle creativity, or we all go down together.

6. **Food and resources must be shared**, and unrestrained population growth curbed to bring us back into balance.

7. **Violence is an archaic and unacceptable way to resolve differences.**

The watchwords are **RESPECT FOR LIFE,
CARE FOR ONE ANOTHER, and
CREATE THE NEW WORLD TOGETHER.**

In these exciting and interesting times, we are called upon to change. This is a change that is demanded of us if we are to survive, and it goes far beyond politics. Everyone knows what direction we need to go, and it is in AMERICA THAT THE GREATEST CHANGE MUST HAPPEN. How will you behave differently? You might start by introducing yourself to your neighbor, or by starting a conversation with a complete stranger. Offer to help someone, do a gratuitous act of kindness. See yourself as a messenger of goodwill and harmony. Listen to others even when they criticize you. What if they're right? Stop taking everything so personally. Learn to live more simply. Make things yourself, instead of buying everything. Involve the kids more; see if you can peel them off the TV or the computer. Shut down electronics completely for a few hours a day. Listen to silence. Walk to the store, or ride a bicycle. Grow something, if only in a window box. Pay attention to life.

It is by simplifying and pulling ourselves back into a sane and sustainable way of life that our personal health will be restored. The concept "natural" should be revered, and plastics and patent medicines used less and less. Take back your space from marketers who bombard you with what you supposedly "need" from them (at a price!). Self-reliance and community connection are empowering and ultimately life-saving. The life you save may be your own, and your children's for generation upon generation.

So the bigger picture of holistic self care includes the need to be a better person, to care for others—even those we don't know personally, or who may not look like us—and the overriding imperative to care for our planet. We must enlist the creative efforts of everyone, reinstate women and the poor to true equality, and balance our desires with the greater good. Then, and only then, will we be truly well. Only then will we be fit to explore the stars and peacefully interact with the life that very likely exists out there.

Afterword

After reading this book, my hope is that you will be inspired to seek out help that is "outside the black bag." Many chiropractors, acupuncture physicians, personal trainers, etc., are very knowledgeable about nutrition. If you have a complex medical problem, please find a physician who has a broader toolbox. This can be a frustrating search in many parts of the country, since holistic physicians are few and far between.

Resources to help you find a holistic doctor are available at:

www.holisticmedicine.org, the website of the American Holistic Medical Association.

www.acam.org, the website of the American College for the Advancement of Medicine. This organization trains doctors in chelation therapy.

www.A4M.com - Anti-aging doctors, knowledgeable in hormone replacement and other techniques of natural age management, are accessible at this site.

Two of the best ways to find a doctor are to ask at your local health food store, and to call a nearby compounding pharmacy. They are sure to know who is prescribing bioidentical hormones in your area.

Remember, even if you have to travel to see one, or pay out-of-pocket, it's worth it to address the real cause of your problem. Don't do "sweeping it under the drug" medicine forever.

Good luck, and God bless!

Index

LaVergne, TN USA
03 September 2010
195750LV00001B/43/P